# Recent Advances in
# Obstetrics & Gynaecology 27

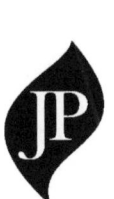

# Recent Advances in
# Obstetrics & Gynaecology 27

**William Ledger** MA DPhil Oxon MB ChB FRCOG FRANZCOG CREI
Professor of Obstetrics and Gynaecology
Royal Hospital for Women
Randwick, Australia

**Justin Clark** MD MRCOG
Consultant
Department of Obstetrics and Gynaecology
Birmingham Women's Hospital
Birmingham, UK

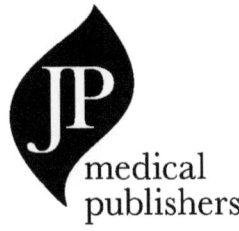

JP
medical
publishers

London • New Delhi

© 2020 Jaypee Brothers Medical Publishers

Published by Jaypee Brothers Medical Publishers,
4838/24 Ansari Road, New Delhi, India

Tel: +91 (011) 43574357          Fax: +91 (011)43574390

Email: info@jpmedpub.com, jaypee@jaypeebrothers.com
Web: www.jpmedpub.com, www.jaypeebrothers.com

JPM is the imprint of Jaypee Brothers Medical Publishers.

The rights of William Ledger and Justin Clark to be identified as the editors of this work have been asserted by them in accordance with the Copyright, Designs and Patents Act 1988.

All rights reserved. No part of this publication may be reproduced, stored or transmitted in any form or by any means, electronic, mechanical, photocopying, recording or otherwise, except as permitted by the UK Copyright, Designs and Patents Act 1988, without the prior permission in writing of the publishers. Permissions may be sought directly from Jaypee Brothers Medical Publishers (P) Ltd. at the address printed above.

All brand names and product names used in this book are trade names, service marks, trademarks or registered trademarks of their respective owners. The publisher is not associated with any product or vendor mentioned in this book.

Medical knowledge and practice change constantly. This book is designed to provide accurate, authoritative information about the subject matter in question. However readers are advised to check the most current information available on procedures included and check information from the manufacturer of each product to be administered, to verify the recommended dose, formula, method and duration of administration, adverse effects and contraindications. It is the responsibility of the practitioner to take all appropriate safety precautions. Neither the publisher nor the authors assume any liability for any injury and/or damage to persons or property arising from or related to use of material in this book.

This book is sold on the understanding that the publisher is not engaged in providing professional medical services. If such advice or services are required, the services of a competent medical professional should be sought.

**ISBN: 978-1-78779-112-1**

**British Library Cataloguing in Publication Data**
A catalogue record for this book is available from the British Library

**Library of Congress Cataloging in Publication Data**
A catalog record for this book is available from the Library of Congress

Development Editor:   Nikita Chauhan
Editorial Assistant:   Keshav Kumar
Cover Design:   Seema Dogra

# Preface

The translation of scientific discovery into clinical practice continues to advance at speed across the diverse range of subspecialties in obstetrics and gynaecology. It is no longer possible for even the most avid of readers to remain abreast of latest developments in all of these areas. It is the purpose of a book of review such as this to help the non-specialists to be updated in some of the most rapidly advancing areas, with chapters written by acknowledged experts and aimed at MRCOG level and above. Our contributors also provide sufficiently detailed information and analysis to interest even those who work in a particular subspecialty – there is always something new, and our authors have been asked to reflect and give their own interpretation of data as well as provide an update on the latest developments. This is the beauty of a review: it is more than a distillation of the clinical science, it imparts to the reader the opinion of the experts in the field on these developments.

The 27th in the series of *Recent Advances in Obstetrics and Gynaecology* maintains the high standards set over many years. It is entertaining to read through the earlier volumes in the series as they reflect changes in thinking and practice over many years. We have moved on in so many ways and yet the basic principles of Medicine as applied in our field remain the same. Our role as doctors is to be professionally empathic, place the patient at the centre at all times, listen and examine carefully and investigate appropriately, thereby selecting the best and least costly treatment for the problem. The authors of the current volume reflect these principles in their articles and provide new insights into the complexities of diagnosis and treatment in our time.

William Ledger
Justin Clark
June 2019

# Contents

| | | |
|---|---|---|
| Preface | | v |
| Chapter 1 | Fetal therapy and surgery<br>*Gulati N, Kilby MD* | 1 |
| Chapter 2 | The impacted head at caesarean section<br>*Annette Briley, Andrew Shennan, Graham Tydeman* | 13 |
| Chapter 3 | Midwifery-led care for women at all levels of risk<br>*Sally K Tracy* | 21 |
| Chapter 4 | The role of urodynamics in female lower urinary tract symptoms<br>*Verghese TS, Latthe P* | 33 |
| Chapter 5 | Medical management of urinary incontinence in the premenopausal woman<br>*Dina El-Hamamsy, Douglas G Tincello* | 45 |
| Chapter 6 | Caesarean scar ectopic pregnancy<br>*Venetia Goodhart* | 57 |
| Chapter 7 | Ambulatory interventions in the management of acute gynaecology and early pregnancy complications<br>*Kim Lawson, Cecilia Bottomley* | 67 |
| Chapter 8 | Hereditary cancer in gynaecology: What clinicians should know about genetic-testing, screening and risk reduction<br>*Faiza Maryam Gaba, Ranjit Manchanda* | 81 |
| Chapter 9 | Vulval cancer in elderly women<br>*Madeleine Macdonald, John Tidy* | 99 |

Content

# Chapter 1

# Fetal therapy and surgery

*Gulati N, Kilby MD*

## INTRODUCTION

Fetal therapy is a rapidly expanding field of medicine and obstetrics, facilitated by advances in imaging, increased understanding of the pathophysiology of diseases, and development of novel therapies to improve perinatal and long-term outcomes of the unborn child.

In utero treatment has the potential to cure or limit disease progression in the fetus, minimise postnatal complications and facilitate therapy in the neonate. Careful patient selection is key as there is a significant risk of maternal morbidity, which must be balanced again the proposed benefit to the fetus. Any advances in treatment techniques must be supported by robust methods to prevent and manage potential complications such as preterm labour and ruptured membranes, which in turn will increase the efficacy of fetal therapies.

Since the first reported human fetal surgery in 1965, fetal therapy has moved from being a purely experimental to an increasingly evidence-based field with systematic reviews and meta-analysis of cohort studies and randomised-controlled trials (RCTs) to support treatment modalities.

To date, there are varying degrees of evidence to support fetal surgery for the following diseases, which will be discussed in turn in this chapter:
- Lower urinary tract obstruction (LUTO)
- Twin-to-twin transfusion syndrome (TTTS)
- Myelomeningocele (MMC)
- Congenital diaphragmatic hernia (CDH)
- Space-occupying lesions such as congenital cystic adenomatoid malformation (CCAM) or sacrococcygeal teratoma (SCT) associated with hydrops
- Selected congenital cardiac abnormalities

Fetal surgery relies upon a multi-disciplinary approach. An experienced team comprising of a fetal medicine specialist, paediatric surgeon, anaesthetist, neonatologist and operating department staff is vital.

---

**Gulati N** BMedSci BMBS MRCOG, Institute of Metabolism & Systems Research, College of Medical Sciences, University of Birmingham and the Fetal Medicine Centre, Birmingham Women's and Children's Foundation Trust, Birmingham, UK

**Kilby MD** MB BS DSc MD FRCOG FRCPI, Institute of Metabolism & Systems Research, College of Medical Sciences, University of Birmingham and the Fetal Medicine Centre, Birmingham Women's and Children's Foundation Trust, Birmingham, UK

There are still many challenges. Understanding of many disease processes remains incomplete and treatments are still imperfect, with significant and potentially unknown long-term effects on the mother and fetus.

Most of the in utero interventions have been made possible because of innovations in 'minimally invasive surgery'; which in this subspecialty involves the use of fetoscopic surgery. It is only the prenatal repair of fetal meningomyelocele that necessitates open fetal surgery and this has not gained widespread use or popularity worldwide. The high-risk nature of these interventions makes it difficult to conduct RCTs, limiting the amount of good-quality evidence available.

# LOWER URINARY TRACT OBSTRUCTION

Fetal vesicoamniotic shunt (VAS) insertion is perhaps one of the most common interventions for LUTO. The aim is to allow fetal urine to pass into the amniotic cavity, allowing an amniotic fluid volume sufficient to theoretically prevent pulmonary hypoplasia (and allow lung development satisfactory for postnatal life). This also allows bypassing of the congenital urethral obstruction and theoretically protects the kidneys from 'damage'. The preferred candidate is a singleton pregnancy with a normal karyotype and an isolated congenital abnormality of congenital bladder neck obstruction or LUTO. This anomaly is actually a heterogeneous group of pathologies; most commonly posterior urethral valves and urethral atresia.

The most common indications for VAS insertion is in congenital bladder neck obstruction (commonly posterior urethral valves) in a male fetus. In female fetuses, more severe forms of LUTO such as urethral atresia tend to be more prevalent, for which VAS insertion is inadequate and more complex intervention is required.

The procedure was first described by Golbus et al. in 1982 [1]. The shunt consists of a pigtail catheter, which is inserted percutaneously via a trocar under ultrasound guidance. The proximal end sits in the fetal bladder and the distal end in the amniotic fluid, thus bypassing the obstruction. The complication rate of VAS insertion is up to 40% [2]. The most common risk of the procedure is miscarriage. However, specific complications related to the procedure include shunt displacement and blockage or the formation of a hernia at the site of shunt entry and bladder rupture. These risks have to be balanced against the poor prognosis associated with conservative management of this congenital abnormality.

Efficacy of VAS insertion has been summarised in a systematic review of cohort studies which showed that antenatal intervention improved perinatal survival compared with no treatment (OR 3.86, 95% CI 2.00 to 7.45) [2]. This effect was particularly significant in the subgroup with poor predicted prognosis on fetal urine sample obtained through a vesicocentesis to analyse fetal renal function pre-intervention. The PLUTO trial was a prospective multicentre RCT to compare long-term outcomes of percutaneous VAS insertion with conservative management [3]. It ended prematurely due to poor recruitment, but the trial demonstrated that of those randomised to VAS, 50% survived to 28 days compared with 27% of those randomised to the conservative management arm. Survival appeared to be higher in the treatment group but direction and magnitude of effect could not be proven conclusively. Regardless of treatment, overall long-term prognosis for all babies was poor; only two babies survived to 2 years of age with normal renal function [1–3].

A longitudinal cohort study of 20 pregnancies affected by LUTO followed up for 5 years showed that surviving male children who underwent VAS insertion in utero were neurodevelopmentally normal and reported normal quality of life. Over half of the group had normal bladder function with spontaneous voiding and 40% had acceptable renal function. One-third required dialysis and transplantation. A significant number of children had persistent respiratory difficulties, musculoskeletal problems including height and weight below the 25th centile, and frequent urinary tract infections [4]. Faced with such mixed outcomes and prognosis, couples often consider termination of pregnancy (TOP) when faced with this diagnosis.

Fetal cystoscopy (the percutaneous ultrasound-guided placement of a 1–2 mm cystoscope into the fetal bladder) may improve the accuracy in correctly diagnosing pathology and has the potential to allow a 'more physiological treatment' of LUTO. Techniques include hydroscopic ablation or laser ablation of any identified posterior urethral valves. Anterograde fetal cystoscopy with maternal and fetal anaesthesia under ultrasound guidance has been shown to have 100% sensitivity and 85.7% specificity for correct diagnosis of LUTO [5]. However, at present, when compared to VAS insertion, therapeutic cystoscopy has no significant improvement in perinatal survival. Large RCTs to compare the two interventions with long-term follow-up of these babies are required.

## TWIN-TO-TWIN TRANSFUSION SYNDROME

Monochorionic pregnancies account for approximately 30% of twin pregnancies in the UK, and rarely, may also occur in higher order pregnancies, particularly triplets (dichorionic or monochorionic). The unique challenge of monochorionic pregnancies stems from the vascular anastomoses in the shared placenta that connect the fetal circulations.

The TTTS complicates up to 15% of monochorionic pregnancies [6]. In this condition, the placentas have predominantly unidirectional arteriovenous anastomoses (AVAs), leading to haemodynamic imbalance between the fetal circulations. This adversely affects fetal cardiac function, renal function and growth, with selective growth restriction occurring in over 50% of monochorionic twins complicated by TTTS [6]. The condition is screened for by ultrasound examination from 16 weeks at 2-weekly intervals until delivery. It is characterised by polyhydramnios (>8 cm prior to 20 weeks and >10 cm after 20 weeks) in the polyuric 'recipient' twin and oligohydramnios (<2 cm) in the oliguric 'donor' twin. It is rare to be diagnosed after 26 weeks gestation. The severity of TTTS is staged using the Quintero system [7]. The prognosis of TTTS is very poor with perinatal mortality being associated with between 90–100% of cases if untreated [6,8].

Traditional (and now historical) treatment options included selective fetocide, serial amnioreduction for maternal symptomatic relief, and amniotic septostomy. These methods, though simpler, had variable survival rates and there is considerable lack of data on long-term morbidity. After proven efficacy in a relatively large RCT, fetoscopic laser coagulation (FLC), was introduced in the 1990s and is the only treatment option which targets the underlying pathology (of unilateral AVAs) and is now the preferred method for management between 16 to 26 weeks of gestation.

FLC involves ultrasound-guided insertion of a 3-mm trocar in to the recipient sac (ideally at right angles to the donor's longitudinal axis) to allow the operator to visualise the intertwin membrane and AVAs. A fetoscope and laser fibre (either an Nd:Yag or diode laser at 40–60 Watts) are introduced through the trocar and anastomoses are coagulated under direct vision. In some cases, amnioinfusion is used to facilitate the procedure, with radical amniodrainage at the end to a normal maximum pool depth (MPD) of ~6 cm. The procedure is conducted under regional or local anaesthesia. Tocolysis and prophylactic antibiotics are commonly used.

Techniques for identifying and selecting vessels to be coagulated include:
- The selective sequential technique – avoiding the AA and VV anastomoses
- The nonselective technique – coagulating all vessels crossing the membrane to ensure none are missed. Missed anastomoses is the most common cause of recurrence and morbidity, with recurrent TTTS occurring in up to 14% of pregnancies treated with FLC and can be associated with or without twin anaemia-polycythaemia sequence (TAPS).
- The equatorial laser dichorionisation (known as the Solomon technique) – this involves completing an initial selective coagulation and then coagulating a dividing line across the vascular equator [8]. There is RCT evidence that this technique reduces the recurrence of TTTS and TAPS compared with the selective sequential technique, such that the Royal College of Obstetricians and Gynaecologists (RCOG) recommends this as the method of choice for FLC [8,9].

A 2014 Cochrane review compared the outcome of FLC with amnioreduction. Although there was no difference in overall death between amnioreduction and laser coagulation (risk ratio (RR) 0.87; 95% confidence interval (CI) 0.55 to 1.38) or death of at least one infant per pregnancy (RR 0.91; 95% CI 0.75 to 1.09), or death of both infants per pregnancy (RR 0.76; 95% CI 0.27 to 2.10), more babies were alive without neurological abnormality at the age of 6 years in the laser group than in the amnioreduction groups (RR 1.57; 95% CI 1.05 to 2.34). There were no significant differences in the babies alive at 6 years with major neurological abnormality treated by laser coagulation or amnioreduction (RR 0.97; 95% CI 0.34 to 2.77) [10].

Overall maternal complication rates of FLC are around 5.4% and include pain secondary to amniotic fluid leaking in to the peritoneal cavity, bleeding, chorioamnionitis and premature, pre-labour rupture of membranes. Abruption and maternal thromboembolism are rare complications. Early fetal complications, which can occur in the first 6 days, include single and double intrauterine death (IUD) and TAPS. Late complications include recurrent or reversed TTTS, late TAPS, IUD (with risks to the surviving twin if single twin demise). Preterm delivery after therapy remains a high risk. Delivery is recommended between $34-36^{+6}$ weeks' gestation though may be considered earlier if there are concerns [8].

Timely referral to a tertiary centre with appropriate expertise is crucial. Morris et al. showed that overall survival following FLC improved after about 61 procedures were performed, and after approximately 3.4 years' experience [11]. As such, it is recommended that centres performing FLC should perform at least 15 procedures each year [8]. Centres will provide FLC to treat Quintero stage II or above TTTS. There is also a case for treatment of stage I TTTS, particularly if there is significant polyhydramnios or cervical shortening [6].

## MYELOMENINGOCELE (OPEN SPINA BIFIDA)

Myelomeningocele is the most common form of spina bifida, characterised by extrusion of the spinal cord in to a sac filled with cerebrospinal fluid (CSF), resulting in life-long disability and neurological dysfunction. Left untreated, babies with the congenital abnormality are born with a degree of damage that cannot be repaired postnatally.

Animal studies have shown that prenatal coverage of a spina bifida lesion preserves neurological function and improves hindbrain herniation, thus supporting a 'two-hit' hypothesis in which the combination of failed neural tube formation and subsequent insult from prolonged exposure of the neurological tissue to the intrauterine environment results in the final deficit [12].

The Management of Myelomeningocele Study (MOMS) RCT compared the safety and efficacy of prenatal repair of MMC with standard postnatal repair and demonstrated that in utero surgery performed before 26 weeks' gestation decreased the risk of death and reduced the need for shunting of CSF by the age of 12 months (40% versus 82% in the postnatal closure group). There was also improved mental and motor function at 30 months of age, reduced incidence of hindbrain herniation, and improved likelihood of being able to walk independently, compared with postnatal surgery. Recruitment was planned for 200 patients but closed after recruitment of 183 because of the clear benefit in the prenatal surgery group [13]. More long-term follow-up of this cohort is awaited and to demonstrate a clear advantage in reduced morbidity in those managed by open fetal surgery.

Repair of MMC is the most common indication for open fetal surgery. Fetoscopic closure has been attempted but so far has not been found to provide as good a surgical result as open repair [14]. However, hysterotomy for open closure carries the life-long risk of uterine rupture from the classical uterine incision, affecting all future pregnancies. Additionally there are the risks of placental abruption, chorioamnionitis, preterm labour as well as the general surgical and anaesthetic risks to consider. Extensive counselling, multidisciplinary planning and appropriate expertise and facilities are crucial and careful patient selection is key. Other anomalies should be excluded and preoperative fetal MRI to assess the level and the extent of the lesion can help to plan the procedure. Operating at earlier gestations ($19–25^{+6}$ weeks) seems to be preferred. Surgery is performed under general anaesthetic, allowing uterine relaxation as well as providing anaesthesia to the mother and fetus. Additional fetal anaesthesia is provided by intramuscular narcotic and neuromuscular blockade prior to fetal incision. Preoperative prophylactic antibiotics and tocolytics are also used to minimise risks. Postoperative maintenance tocolysis may also be used to reduce the risk of preterm labour [13,14].

Long-term outcomes of babies who have undergone open fetal surgery are yet to be fully assessed to determine whether the benefits demonstrated by the MOMS in early childhood years are worth the maternal and fetal risks of the surgery.

There are also cohort series describing fetoscopically-assisted MMC surgical management. If the time of surgery can be reduced then this would seem a more attractive option for surgical management than open hysterotomy.

## CONGENITAL DIAPHRAGMATIC HERNIA

Congenital diaphragmatic hernia (CDH) is a condition in which the abdominal viscera herniate through the diaphragm in to the mediastinum, causing significantly impaired development of the lungs. Whilst CDH itself is surgically correctable, pulmonary hypoplasia can affect fitness for surgery and can mean that neonates die before surgery can be done. The aim of in utero treatment is to minimise pulmonary hypoplasia and therefore attempt to improve the prognosis in postnatal life.

There is some experimental evidence suggesting that open fetal surgery to repair CDH in utero is feasible in those without liver herniation (in utero fetal repair for those with liver herniation would occlude the umbilical vein) [15]. However, these feasibility studies showed that there was no difference in survival between those who underwent fetal surgery and those who received standard postnatal management. Additionally, the fetal surgery patients were born more prematurely and required as much ventilatory support as the postnatal intervention group [15].

Fetoscopic endoluminal tracheal occlusion (FETO) appears to show promise in case cohort studies [16]. Fetuses will still require neonatal repair of the hernia, however, animal models have demonstrated that FETO will trigger lung growth by preventing lung fluid from escaping, creating a positive pressure to stent and distend the lungs and therefore encourage alveoli formation and subsequently increase the lung surface area [17]. The procedure is done percutaneously via a trocar under regional and local anaesthetic at 26-28 weeks' gestation [18]. The balloon is able to accommodate for the increasing tracheal diameter as the fetus grows. The aim is to then puncture the balloon under ultrasound-guidance or remove it fetoscopically at 34 weeks to enable further lung maturation. Traditionally, the balloon had been removed at the time of caesarean section (CS) by ex-utero intrapartum therapy (EXIT). However, removing the balloon in utero facilitates vaginal delivery and has been associated with a better lung maturation in animal studies [17,18].

Initial European collaborative trials have shown the benefits of FETO over conservative antenatal management [16]. A series of 210 cases with a median delivery gestation of 35.3 weeks demonstrated that in 97.1% of cases the babies were born alive and 48% were discharged home from hospital alive. The study estimated that the survival rate for left CDH treated with FETO increased from 24.1% to 49.1% and from 0% to 35.3% in right CDH ($P$ <0.001) [16]. Predictors for survival include the observed/expected lung area to head circumference ratio (o/e LHR) prior to the procedure, and the gestational age at delivery [19].

This minimally invasive approach avoids the complications of laparotomy and hysterotomy associated with an open technique. However, iatrogenic preterm prelabour rupture of membranes (PPROM) occurred in 47.1% of cases at 3-83 days postprocedure in the aforementioned case series and within 3 weeks in 16.7% of cases [16]. Ten babies died as a direct result of difficulties removing the balloon and hence a unique dilemma with FETO is unplanned removal of the balloon in an emergency setting [16,19,20].

Nevertheless a subsequent RCT in Brazil has reproduced the results of the European collaborative studies and shown that FETO improves neonatal survival in cases with severe isolated CDH (RR 10.0, CI 1.4-70.6, $P$ <0.01) despite a lower mean gestational age at delivery (35.6 ± 2.4 weeks versus 37.4 ± 1.9 weeks) [21].

Further trials are currently ongoing and results are widely anticipated in order move this from an experimental to an evidence-based form of fetal therapy.

## CONGENITAL LUNG LESIONS

Congenital cystic adenomatoid malformation and bronchopulmonary sequestrations (BPSs) are the most common forms of congenital lung lesions. The incidence of CCAM has been reported to be between 1/25,000 and 1/35,000 live births [22].

The CCAM is described as an overgrowth of terminal respiratory bronchioles that form cysts. It has been postulated that the *Hoxb-5* gene, which is thought to play a role in controlling airway patterning, is abnormally expressed in BPS and CCAM, and therefore associated with abnormal lung tissue development [23].

The cysts are classified by appearance on ultrasound as either macrocystic (containing at least one cyst >5 mm) or microcystic, showing no cysts and appear echogenic. BPS consists of nonfunctioning lung tissue without communication of the bronchopulmonary tree and have an anomalous arterial blood supply. They can be seen on ultrasound as an echodense homogenous mass that may appear similar to a microcystic CCAM lesion. However, BPS may be differentiated by colour flow Doppler which demonstrates arterial blood flow from the aorta directly to the BPS mass, though this differentiation is not always possible antenatally [24].

Whilst microcystic lesions often regress spontaneously after a peak growth at 26–28 weeks, macrocystic lesions do not regress because of continued fluid accumulation in the cyst and will require postnatal follow-up and likely definitive surgery to reduce the risk of infection or malignancy [25,26]. Very large or rapidly expanding large lesions will cause significant compression of lung tissue leading to pulmonary hypoplasia and fetal hydrops secondary to a mass effect causing mediastinal shift, vena caval compression and impaired cardiac function [24]. It is this rare subset that may benefit from fetal surgery. The prognosis of expectantly managed CCAM with fetal hydrops is extremely poor with studies reporting survival at 0–3% compared with nonhydropic fetuses at 97.6–100% survival [25,26].

Serial thoracocentesis, thoracoamniotic shunt placement and open fetal surgery have all been described as methods to facilitate normal lung development and reduce the mass effect. There are no RCTs available to compare intervention with conservative management or to determine the best mode of treatment, however there are a number of observational studies describing outcomes of thoracoamniotic shunts in macrocystic pulmonary lesions. The procedure and complications are the same as for VAS insertion, with the pigtail catheter being inserted under ultrasound guidance into the lower pleural cavity, posterior to the midaxillary line. In one retrospective review [24], shunts were inserted at a mean gestational age of 24.6 in 11 cases with very large macrocystic lesions and mediastinal shift. Six of these were hydropic, of which three also had polyhydramnios. Of the nonhydropic fetuses, the lesions were either growing very rapidly in size, had large CCAM volume ratios at initial presentation (this fetus died at 17 weeks' gestation, 1 day after shunt insertion), had marked polyhydramnios or had rapidly reaccumulating cysts with evolving hydrops despite serial thoracocentesis. Shunting of one cyst decompressed the entire lesion in every fetus, indicating communication between the cysts. Hydrops and/or polyhydramnios resolved in all affected cases. The babies were delivered vaginally at term, with no maternal morbidity. All newborns underwent uneventful lobectomies. Overall reported survival of hydropic fetuses after shunt insertion is approximately two-thirds.

Whilst there is support for this procedure for large macrocystic CCAM with mediastinal shift and hydrops, in which the prognosis if left untreated is very poor, there is controversy regarding intervention for nonhydropic fetuses, mainly due to a lack of evidence that there is any significant difference in survival in those treated versus those left untreated, and difficulty in predicting whether these lesions will grow or resolve spontaneously, which many do. In cases with microcystic CCAM and hydrops, there is some evidence to suggest open fetal surgery with in utero lobectomy may improve survival, though this is at significant risk to the mother [24].

There is a real need for good quality trials to evaluate treatment of fetal lung lesions, though initial evidence seems favourable for the most severely affected fetuses.

## SACROCOCCYGEAL TERATOMA

Fetal SCT occur in 1–2 per 20,000 pregnancies. Perinatal mortality of those lesions diagnosed antenatally is between 25–37%. However fast growing, solid and highly vascularised lesions can cause high-output cardiac failure and present clinically with polyhydramnios, hydrops and IUD. Mortality for this subset of fetuses is close to 100% [27]. Hydrops with SCT can also cause maternal 'mirror' syndrome – a rare, severe form of pre-eclampsia. There are a few case series which describe different surgical procedures. Open fetal surgery may improve survival but is associated with substantial risks to mother and fetus. Attempts at minimally invasive procedures include fetoscopic laser ablation of tumour vessels, similar to the approach for treatment of TTTS, radiofrequency ablation, and thrombogenic coiling. Survival rates following minimally invasive procedures are reported at 30%, and up to 55% for open surgery [27]. Complications of these procedures include IUD, PPROM and preterm labour, although long-term outcomes of these fetal surgeries have yet to be reported. Mean gestational age at delivery has been reported at 30 weeks [27]. Intraoperative deaths associated with the minimally invasive techniques have occurred secondary to rupture of the tumour or bleeding in to the tumour, and so there is an argument for optimising haemoglobin levels preoperatively with intrauterine transfusion if necessary [27]. Minimally invasive techniques can also cause collateral damage to the fetal perineum. As the disease is rare, it would be difficult to conduct an RCT with adequate recruitment; however, current literature suggests that fetal intervention may have some benefit in selected cases suffering significant effects from the SCT [27]. Nevertheless, fetal therapy for this congenital abnormality is still very much experimental and limited to highly-trained and experienced fetal medicine specialists.

## CONGENITAL CARDIAC ABNORMALITIES

The current literature describes in utero treatment for a number of congenital cardiac diseases, with varying successes and outcomes.

Intrauterine balloon valvuloplasty for critical aortic stenosis has been reported as a means of preventing hypoplastic left heart syndrome at 21–29 weeks' gestation with a technical success rate of 70% [28]. A case series of 24 fetuses with critical aortic stenosis who underwent ultrasound-guided transabdominal valvuloplasty showed that 66.7% had a biventricular circulation postnatally and regression of hydrops in those that were affected (17%) [29].

Pulmonary atresia with an intact ventricular septum and evolving hypoplastic right heart syndrome has been treated in limited cases with ultrasound guided pulmonary balloon valvuloplasty in the second trimester. Access to the right ventricular outflow tract is through direct puncture in to the fetal chest wall either subcostally or in the intercostal space lateral to the sternum [28]. Intervention in these select cases demonstrated an improved circulation and more substantial right heart structures compared with controls [30].

Hypoplastic left heart syndrome with an intact or tight atrial septum may cause pulmonary oedema and pulmonary hypertension postnatally if left untreated. In utero ultrasound-guided balloon atrial septostomy may minimise the effects of the anomaly on the pulmonary vasculature. In some cases, a stent can be placed across the septum following septostomy to prevent closure [28]. Sadly the procedure is yet to show any benefit on postnatal outcomes as mortality remains high in spite of fetal therapy, and numbers are too small.

However, an International Consortium of Fetal Cardiology Therapists are starting to pool their results and publish their data in the public domain for critical appraisal [31].

Fetal bradycardia due to complete fetal heart block (associated with maternal anti-Rho and La antibodies) has been treated in select cases with in utero placement of a cardiac pacemaker when medical therapies have failed. A single-chamber pacing system can be placed on to the fetal myocardium either transcutaneously via ultrasound or fetoscopically. Dislodgement of the leads from fetal movements has limited the success of this intervention [28].

The above procedures are still very much at an experimental stage. Careful patient selection, development of more sophisticated techniques and trials are crucial to improving outcome and ensuring perceived benefits outweigh procedure risks.

# SUMMARY

Fetal surgery is an ever-evolving area within obstetrics and gynaecology. Patient willingness to participate in experimental therapies opens the gateway to trial novel strategies for treating otherwise fatal or severely debilitating fetal conditions. This has to be supported by a continuous multidisciplinary discussion about the suitability of any proposed procedure and the risks involved to mother and/or fetus. Case series, feasibility studies and RCTs are helping to bring this subspecialist area on to an evidence-based platform.

> **Key points for clinical practice**
> 
> - Fetal therapy is a rapidly expanding field, facilitated by advances in imaging, increased knowledge of diseases and development of novel therapies.
> - Lower urinary tract obstruction caused by posterior urethral valves has been treated with vesicoamniotic shunts with varying success on long-term follow-up.
> - TTTS affects 30% of monochorionic twin pregnancies. Fetoscopic laser ablation has been shown to result in more babies surviving without neurological abnormalities at the age of 6 compared with amnioreduction.
> - Myelomeningocele is currently the most common indication for open fetal surgery and via RCT has been shown to provide a better neurological outcome than postnatal surgery, though this needs to be balanced with maternal risks including uterine scarring.
> - Congenital diaphragmatic hernias have been successfully managed with fetoscopic endoluminal tracheal occlusion to facilitate lung development. However, deaths have occurred as a direct result of difficulty removing the balloon and so it is vital that services conducting this procedure have 24/7 availability in case unplanned removal is required.
> - Congenital cystic adenomatoid malformation and bronchopulmonary sequestrations are rare, however very large lesions cause pulmonary hypoplasia and mediastinal shift, leading to hydrops. Thoracoamniotic shunting has been shown to benefit this small subset of affected fetuses. Management of microcystic lesions and stable lesions without hydrops is more controversial as many will be self-limiting or regress.
> - Sacrococcygeal teratomas associated with cardiac failure and hydrops has a perinatal mortality close to 100%. Various minimally invasive procedures have been experimented to interrupt the blood supply to these tumours with limited success.
> - Congenital cardiac diseases including critical aortic stenosis, pulmonary atresia, hypoplastic left heart with a closed ventricular septum and heart block have all been experimentally treated by minimally invasive techniques although statistically significant benefits are yet to be seen.

## REFERENCES

1. Golbus MS, Harrison M, Filly RA, et al. In utero treatment of urinary tract obstruction. Am J Obstet Gynecol 1982; 142:383–388.
2. Morris RK, Malin GL, Khan KS, Kilby MD. Systematic review of the effectiveness of antenatal intervention for the treatment of congenital lower urinary tract obstruction. BJOG 2010; 117:382–390.
3. Morris RK, Malin GL, Quinlan-Jones E, et al. for the Percutaneous vesicoamniotic shunting in Lower Urinary Tract Obstruction (PLUTO) Collaborative Group. Percutaneous vesicoamniotic shunting versus conservative management for fetal lower urinary tract obstruction (PLUTO): a randomised trial. Lancet 2013; 382:1496–1506.
4. Biard JM, Johnson MP, Carr MC, et al. Long-term outcomes in children treated by prenatal vesicoamniotic shunting for lower urinary tract obstruction. Obstet Gynecol 2005; 106:503–508.
5. Malin G, Tonks AM, Morris RK, et al. Congenital lower urinary tract obstruction: a population-based epidemiological study. BJOG 2012; 119:1455–1464.
6. Kilby MD, Baker PN, Critchley HO, et al. Consensus views arising from the 50th Study Group: Multiple Pregnancy. Multiple Pregnancy. London: RCOG Press 2006:283–286.
7. Quintero RA, Morales WJ, Allen MH, et al. Staging of twin-twin transfusion syndrome. J Perinatol 1999; 19:550–555.
8. Kilby MD, Bricker L on behalf of the Royal College of Obstetricians and Gynaecologists. Management of monochorionic twin pregnancy. BJOG 2016; 124:e1–e45.
9. Slaghekke F, Lopriore E, Lewi L, et al. Fetoscopic laser coagulation of the vascular equator versus selective coagulation for twin-to-twin transfusion syndrome: an open-label randomised controlled trial. Lancet 2014; 383:2144–2151.
10. Roberts D, Neilson JP, Kilby MD, Gates S. Interventions for the treatment of twin-twin transfusion syndrome. Cochrane Database Syst Rev 2014:CD002073.
11. Morris RK, Selman TJ, Harbidge A, et al. Fetoscopic laser coagulation for severe twin-to-twin transfusion syndrome: factors influencing perinatal outcome, learning curve of the procedure and lessons for new centres. BJOG 2010; 117:1350–1357.
12. Bouchard S, Davey MG, Rintoul NE, et al. Correction of hindbrain herniation and anatomy of the vermis following in utero repair of myelomeningocele in sheep. J Pediatr Surg 2003; 38:451–458.
13. Adzick NS, Thom EA, Spong CY, et al. A randomized trial of prenatal versus postnatal repair of myelomeningocele. N Engl J Med 2011; 364:993–1004.
14. Farmer DL, von Koch CS, Peacock WJ, et al. In utero repair of myelomeningocele: experimental pathophysiology, initial clinical experience, and outcomes. Arch Surg 2003; 138:872–878.
15. Harrison MR, Adzick NS, Bullard KM, et al. Correction of congenital diaphragmatic hernia in utero VII: a prospective trial. J Pediatr Surg 1997; 32:1637–1642.
16. Jani JC, Nicolaides KH, Gratacós E, et al. Severe diaphragmatic hernia treated by fetal endoscopic tracheal occlusion. Ultrasound Obstet Gynecol 2009; 34:304–310.
17. Flageole H, Evrard V, Piedboeuf B, et al. The plug-unplug sequence: an important step to achieve type II pneumocyte maturation in the fetal lamb model. J Pediatr Surg 1998; 33:299–303.
18. Deprest J, Nicolaides K, Done' E, et al. Technical aspects of fetal endoscopic tracheal occlusion for congenital diaphragmatic hernia. J Pediatr Surg 2011; 46:22–32.
19. Jani JC, Nicolaides KH, Gratacos E, et al. Fetal lung-to-head ratio in the prediction of survival in severe left-sided diaphragmatic hernia treated by fetal endoscopic tracheal occlusion (FETO). Am J Obstet Gynecol 2006; 195:1646–1650.
20. Deprest J, Nicolaides K, Gratacós E. Fetal surgery for congenital diaphragmatic hernia is back from never gone. Fetal Diagn Therapy 2011; 29:6–17.
21. Ruano R, Yoshisaki CT, da Silva MM, et al. A randomized controlled trial of fetal endoscopic tracheal occlusion versus postnatal management of severe isolated congenital diaphragmatic hernia. Ultrasound Obstet Gynecol 2012; 39:20–27.
22. Laberge JM, Flageole H, Pugash D, et al. Outcome of the prenatally diagnosed congenital cystic adenomatoid lung malformation: a Canadian experience. Fetal Diagn Ther 2001; 16:178–186.
23. Volpe MV, Pham L, Lessin M, et al. Expression of Hoxb-5 during human lung development and in congenital lung malformations. Birth Defects Res A Clin Mol Teratol 2003; 67:550–556.
24. Schrey S, Kelly EN, Langer JC, et al. Fetal thoracoamniotic shunting for large macrocystic congenital cystic adenomatoid malformations of the lung. Ultrasound Obstet Gynecol 2012; 39:515–520.

25. Adzick NS, Harrison MR, Crombleholme TM, et al. Fetal lung lesions: management and outcome. Am J Obstet Gynecol 1998; 179:884–889.
26. Davenport M, Warne SA, Cacciaguerra S, et al. Current outcome of antenally diagnosed cystic lung disease. J Pediatr Surg 2004; 39:549–556.
27. Mieghem TV, Al-Ibrahim A, Deprest J, et al. Minimally invasive therapy for fetal sacrococcygeal teratoma: case series and systematic review of the literature. Ultrasound Obstet Gynecol 2014; 43:611–619.
28. Yuan S. Fetal cardiac interventions: an update of therapeutic options. Rev Bras Cir Cardiovasc 2014; 29:388–395.
29. Arzt W, Wertaschnigg D, Veit I, et al. Intrauterine aortic valvuloplasty in fetuses with critical aortic stenosis: experience and results of 24 procedures. Ultrasound Obstet Gynecol 2011; 37:689–695.
30. Tworetzky W, McElhinney DB, Marx GR, et al. In utero valvuloplasty for pulmonary atresia with hypoplastic right ventricle: techniques and outcomes. Pediatrics 2009; 124:e510–518.
31. Moon-Grady AJ, Morris SA, Belfort M. International Fetal Cardiac Intervention Registry: A Worldwide Collaborative Description and Preliminary Outcomes. J Am Coll Cardiol 2015; 66:388–399.

# Chapter 2

# The impacted head at caesarean section

*Annette Briley, Andrew Shennan, Graham Tydeman*

## THE SIZE OF THE PROBLEM

Caesarean section (CS) rates in the UK vary from 26% in Wales to 31.1% in Scotland (England 27.1%; Northern Ireland 29.9%) [1].

With total births in 2015 reaching 760,845 it can be estimated that 228,250 babies were born by CS. Elective operations occur in 14-15% of all births [1]. Therefore, more than 105,000 occurred as emergencies, some of which were undertaken late in the first or second stage of labour, when the fetal head has descended low in the maternal pelvis.

The proportion of CS undertaken in the second stage of labour is projected to increase for several reasons. These include: a decline in the use of rotational and midcavity forceps deliveries; an overall decline in assisted vaginal births; a move towards vacuum births, known to have a higher failure rate and increased use of regional analgesia with concomitant prolongation of the second stage. These factors, combined with increasing prevalence of maternal obesity and fetal macrosomia, are likely to further contribute to a rising incidence of impacted fetal head [2].

During CS in late labour the surgeon has to reach deep into the woman's pelvis and gain access below the fetal head in order to lift it out and deliver the baby. In late labour, the fetal head can become impacted between the maternal bony pelvis and soft tissues, causing difficulty in obtaining access below the head. Even when access is achieved, there may be further difficulty in overcoming the partial vacuum that forms beneath the baby's head. Despite second stage CS becoming more common [3] the incidence of difficulty in delivering the fetal head is largely unknown, although Loudon and colleagues reported 30% of emergency CS undertaken in late labour recorded difficulty in delivering the fetal head [4]. Data currently in press from one maternity provider in Scotland reported some degree of difficulty in delivering the fetal head in 18% of all emergency CS (81/440). This was most common when cervical dilatation was ≥8 cm (124/440; 48%), but was also seen at lower dilatations (21/440; 6.5%) [5]. It is reasonable

---

**Annette Briley** PhD MSc RM, Consultant midwife and clinical trials manager Kings College London Division of Women's Health, London, UK

**Andrew Shennan** MBBS MD FRCOG, Professor of Obstetrics Kings College London Division of Women's Health, London, UK

**Graham Tydeman** BSc MBBCh FRCOG, Consultant in O+G, NHS Fife, Kirkcaldy, UK

to state that impaction of the fetal head is a recognised complication encountered by most labour ward clinicians.

## IMPLICATIONS

Impaction of the fetal head at CS has been associated with maternal and neonatal morbidities [3]. Neonatal morbidities most commonly reported are localised bruising and lacerations to the face and head. These may be considered relatively minor, but have implications for increased risk of jaundice requiring phototherapy, and irritability, leading to prolongation of hospital stay, difficulty in establishing breastfeeding, and inherent longer term bonding issues. More serious but less common neonatal complications include neonatal hypoxia, skull fractures, haematomas, brachial plexus injuries, seizures and increased incidence of neonatal unit admissions [6–8]; all of which could have longer term health implications for the child.

Difficulty in delivering the impacted fetal head has been associated with a 36% increase in measured maternal blood loss and is also associated with bladder trauma; wound infection; uterine tears; haematoma and longer hospital stays [9,10]. There is a paucity of data regarding longer-term outcomes but the Birth Trauma Association (BTA) report multiple morbidities including incontinence, prolapse, dyspareunia, fistula, anal sphincter injury and post-traumatic stress disorder.

This clinical emergency also impacts on staff. Due to the unpredictability of the situation, many junior doctors will encounter difficulty in delivering an impacted fetal head out of hours when senior assistance may be unavailable. Midwives and other allied health professionals are often asked to assist and many feel uncertain about the pressure to apply and uncomfortable about undertaking this during surgery.

## CURRENT GUIDELINES

There are currently no national guidelines recommending a single technique to deal with this situation, and a range of techniques are employed. The National Institute for Health and Clinical Excellence (NICE) states that techniques used are associated with maternal and neonatal trauma and there is currently inadequate evidence available to recommend inserting a balloon device to disimpact the deeply engaged fetal head at CS [11].

The Cochrane review, undertaken in 2016 [7], concluded that reverse breech extraction may be associated with less neonatal morbidity than the push method, which involves elevation through pressure applied to the fetal head via the vagina. This may have been due to the impact of studies from low and middle resource settings. Certainly, a survey of trainees in the UK and an audit in one NHS provider found that the push method was universally used [5,9]. Both concluded that more work in the area is required.

## TECHNIQUES DESCRIBED IN THE LITERATURE TO FACILITATE DELIVERY OF THE IMPACTED FETAL HEAD

### Patwardhan's technique

First described in 1957 [12] it is still advocated by some.

It is only relevant when the deeply engaged fetal head is either occipito-transverse (OT) or occipito-anterior (OA).

In these cases, an incision is made in the lower uterine segment, at the level of the anterior shoulder, which is delivered first.

Using gentle traction on the shoulder, the posterior shoulder is delivered.

The surgeon then hooks his fingers through both axillae and using gentle traction, aided by an assistant providing fundal pressure, the body of the fetus is brought out of the uterus.

Only the baby's head remains in the uterus and this is gently lifted out of the pelvis.

Evaluation of this technique has been undertaken in one retrospective case review study ($n = 79$) and another prospective cohort ($n = 50$) in developing countries and reported less incidence of maternal and neonatal morbidities than either the push or the pull method [13,14]. Additionally, impaction of the head would need to be anticipated for this technique to be used, and whilst this may be more predictable in developing countries, where many women transfer for delivery following many hours laboring elsewhere, in the UK situation prediction of difficulty in delivering the fetal head remains challenging.

## Shazly's step

Described in 2013 in a case series of eight patients, this technique involves abdominal disimpaction with lower segment support as a novel technique to minimise moridities [15]. The edge of the lower uterine segment is grasped with forceps applied approximately 2 cm apart along the lower edge of the incision, until it is completely supported. These forceps are handled by an assistant and gentle upward traction, perpendicular to the uterine surface, is applied. There is now adequate space for the surgeon's hand to undertake manipulation without applying pressure on the lower segment, and the fetal head can be delivered. The authors describe it as a promising technique to minimise complications during CS for obstructed labour. However no further investigations have been undertaken, although a research protocol has been registered (ClinicalTrials.gov ID: NCT02934516) to compare this technique with the 'classic' push method. Ethics review is pending and recruitment is anticipated to commence late 2017/early 2018 [16].

## Push method

The push method of cephalic replacement has been the favoured technique in the UK and USA since the 1980s.

The woman is placed into a frog-legged position with knees flexed and thighs abducted. Using an aseptic technique an assistant inserts a hand into the vagina and using cupped fingers gently pushes the fetal head superiorly into the pelvis. At the same time, the surgeon applies traction to the fetal shoulders or attempts to flex and elevate the fetal head [17].

Some clinicians practice a bimanual push method whereby the surgeon elevates the fetal head with a hand from below whilst simultaneously elevating the head with the other hand in the uterus [18].

## Reverse breech extraction (The "pull' method)

This is more widely used in developing countries but many UK based clinicians who have not worked overseas, have not seen this technique.

With this method the surgeon reaches upwards the upper uterine segment and holds one or both fetal legs. Gentle traction is applied until the second leg is apparent. Both fetal legs are delivered by gentle traction (similar to a footling breech technique). During this procedure a low transverse incision may require extension into an inverse T or J-shaped wound to maximise space [19].

## EVIDENCE COMPARING TECHNIQUES

A Cochrane review investigating techniques for assisting with delivery of the impacted fetal head included four trials (357 women) compared the push method versus the pull method. In three studies (239 women), the primary outcome was birth trauma for the infant and there was no difference with either technique for this relatively rare outcome (risk ratio 1.55 95% CI 0.42 to 5.73), although the small sample size may not show clinically important effects. There were also no differences for many secondary outcomes (blood loss > 500 mL, blood transfusion, wound infection, mean hospital stay, Apgar scores). Heterogeneity between trials confounded comparison but the duration of operation was significantly shorter for reverse breech extraction, which may contribute to fewer adverse maternal outcomes in this group [7].

The authors concluded that whilst there is limited evidence that reverse breech may improve maternal and fetal outcomes there was no difference in infant birth trauma and further randomised trials are needed to investigate this further [7].

The use of tocolytics to relax the uterus and therefore make it easier to deliver the infant where difficulty is anticipated was also reviewed. However, the authors concluded that the single randomised trial (97 women) in the literature did not provide sufficient evidence to support or refute this practice [7].

An earlier meta-analysis included 11 studies (1028 women), prospective and retrospective, and incorporating a variety of delivery techniques, reported increased rates of wound extensions, greater blood loss and transfusion and longer operating time in the push group. However there were three long bone fractures in the infant in the pull group compared to none in the push group. All included studies were undertaken in non-Western and non-European settings so the generalisability of the findings is limited [20].

## DEVICES DEVELOPED TO ASSIST WITH DELIVERY OF THE IMPACTED FETAL HEAD

### Murless head extractor

Developed in South Africa in the 1940s this single blade device was first used in the UK in the 1950s [21]. Initial evaluation in the US used the device on 40 unselected women undergoing. The authors found the device expedited delivery in all cases but was particularly useful when the head was deeply engaged in the pelvis [22]. Further evaluation occurred in 1992 when it was similarly deemed useful and not associated with increased maternal or neonatal morbidities [23].

Although still available, there is no evidence in the literature of recent use of this device.

### C-Snorkel

This is a sterile, molded polymer tube with an internal diameter of approximately 1 cm. Inserted vaginally and placed close to the fetal head, this tube facilitates the passage of air around the head, thus overcoming the partial vacuum that has formed making it easier for the surgeon to place a hand beneath the head and deliver it. In a small study ($n = 23$), the device was compared with 49 retrospectively selected cases, where it was not used. The effectiveness of the device was dependent on the station of the fetal head during surgery with fewer hysterotomy extensions at mid-cavity ($n = 0/17$ versus $n = 14/41$, 34%, $P <0.01$) and fewer push-ups required ($n = 0/17$ versus $n = 11/41$, 27% $P = 0.02$). These differences were not seen when the presenting part was at a low station (+2, +3) and indeed confirmation of this significant difference requires confirmation in a robust randomised controlled trial (RCT). The device was positively reviewed by junior staff but there was little consensus amongst senior colleagues regarding its utility [24].

## Fetal Pillow

Safe Obstetric Systems have developed the Fetal Pillow. This device is formed of a foldable baseplate with an attached silicone balloon and a thin tube, with a two-way connector. The baseplate and balloon are inserted vaginally and once in place between the perineal muscles and the fetal head, inflated with 180 mL saline. The aim of the device is to elevate the fetal head to facilitate easier delivery with minimal manipulation. The device is deflated postoperatively via the two way connector and removed by gently pulling the tubing. An initial prospective observational study with historical controls reported an average 4 cm elevation of the fetal head was achieved in all cases ($n = 50$). Additionally, compared with the control group, there were fewer uterine extensions in the fetal pillow group ($P = 0.03$), incision to delivery interval was shorter ($P <0.001$) as were hospital stay ($P \leq 0.001$). There was no statistical difference between groups for blood loss >1,000 mL, blood transfusions, maternal deaths or admission to ITU [25]. Subsequently, the same authors undertook a RCT to further evaluate the device. This larger study ($n = 240$) devised a grading system for uterine extensions and used major, defined as grades 2–3 as the primary endpoint for the study, which were less common in the fetal pillow group. Other outcomes included less blood loss >1,000 mL fewer transfusions. For the neonate there was a reduction in both admissions to NICU and stays >24 hours, but these failed to reach statistical significance [26].

Both these studies were wholly [25] or partially [26] commercially sponsored, and independent verification of these promising results is required given the cost of the device.

## Tydeman tube

The Tydeman tube has been developed to overcome both the partially formed vacuum as well as assist elevation of the impacted fetal head, following established principles of the push technique but using a device designed to reduce trauma and ease the procedure. It is made of silicone and consists of two parts; the cup which is soft and is inserted into the vagina to lie against the fetal head. It is attached to a slightly curved, semi rigid wide-bore tube, which allows air to enter from below. Should a push up be required this can be done from outside the mother's body with the cup applying the force to the baby's head over a larger area than is possible with manual elevation. Tests on a simulator, have shown that greater elevation is achieved with the Tydeman tube compared with digital elevation (mean difference +9.1 mm $P <0.001$), and that although greater force was applied to achieve this (mean difference +0.42 Kgf, $P <0.001$) the force was spread over 6.97 cm$^2$ versus 2.0 cm$^2$ and therefore is may be less likely to cause fetal damage [27]. These authors also reported a case series of the first 10 Tydeman Tubes used in clinical practice. All devices were used in nulliparous women with cervical dilatation 9 cm or 10 cm. All Apgar scores were >8 at 1 and

5 minutes. In one case, the Tydeman tube was only used as elevation could not be achieved with a digital technique.

The mean score for all operators was 7.7/10 suggesting that clinicians found the device easy to use.

Further evaluation of the device in clinical trials is planned.

## CONCLUSION

Difficulty in delivering the fetal head at CS in late labour is not uncommon. In some situations, it can be predicted but often it is unexpected. Although various techniques and devices are available, there are currently no guidelines as to how best to deal with this obstetric emergency, with most clinicians relying on advice and experience of those around them. Given current strategies to prevent primary CS, and changes in maternal demography and staff training, the incidence of impaction of the fetal head is likely to increase.

The lack of evidence around best practice to deal with this is well reported and the need for further research outlined [7,10].

## REFERENCES

1. Office of National Statistics. Hospital Maternity Activity 2015-2016 www.content.digital.nhs.uk 2016. Downloaded 02/05/2017.
2. Manning JB, Tolcher MC, Chandraharan E, Rose CH. Delivery of an impacted fetal head during cesarean: A literature review and proposed management algorithm. Obstet Gynecol Surv 2015; 70:719–724.
3. Unterschieider J, McMenamin M, Cullinane F. Rising rates of caesarean deliveries at full cervical dilatation: a concerning trend. Eur J Obstet Gynecol Reprod Biol 2011; 157:141–144.
4. Loudon JA, Groom KM, Hinkson D, Patterson-Brown S. Changing trends in operative delivery performed at full dilatation over a 10-year period. J Obstet Gynaecol 2010; 30:370–375.
5. Rice A. Incidence of impacted head at caesarean section (CS): PL.38 Journals@Ovid Full TextBJOG. Int J Obstet Gynaecol 2015; 122:88.
6. Asicioglu O, Gungorduk K, Yildrim G, et al. Second-stage vs first-stage caesarean delivery: comparison of maternal and perinatal outcomes. J Obstet Gynaecol 2014; 34:598–504.
7. Waterfall H, Grivell R, Dodd JM. Techniques for assisting difficult delivery at caesarean section. Cochrane Database Syst Rev 2016:CD004944.
8. Mckelvey A, Ashe R, McKenna D, Roberts D. Caesarean section in the second stage of labour: a retrospective review of obstetric setting and morbidity. J Obstet Gynaecol 2010; 30:264–267.
9. Jeve YB, Navti OB, Konje JC. Comparison of techniques used to deliver a deeply impacted fetal head at full dilatation: a systematic review and meta-analysis. BJOG 2016; 123:337–345.
10. Allen VM, O'Connell CM, Baskett TF. Maternal and perinatal morbidity of caesarean delivery at full dilatation compared with caesarean delivery in the first stage of labour. BJOG 2005; 112:986–990.
11. National Institute for health and Clinical Excellence. Insertion of a balloon device to disimpact an engaged fetal head before an emergency caesarean section. NICE 2015; IPG515.
12. Patwardhan BD, Motashaw ND. Caesarean section. J Obstet Gynecol India 1957; 8:1–15.
13. Saha PK, Gulati R, Goel P, Tandon R, Huria A. Second stage caesarean section: evaluation of the patwardhan technique. J Clin Diagn Res 2014; 8:93–95.
14. Mahapatra M. Patwardan's technique: impact on maternal and fetal outcome. YUVA J Med Sci 2015; 1:26–27.
15. Shazly SAM, Elsayed AH, Badran SMA, Abdel Badee AY, Ali MK. Abdominal disimpaction with lower uterine segment support as a novel technique to minimize fetal and maternal morbidities during cesarean section for obstructed labor: a case series. Am J Perinatol 2013; 30:695–698.
16. Abbas AM, Nasr A, Shazly SAM. Delivery of impacted fetal head during cesarean section for obstructed labor: Push method versus abdominal disimpaction with lower uterine segment support (PLUS). ClinicalTrials.giv PRS, 2016.

17. Landesman R, Graber EA. Abdominovaginal delivery: modifications of the cesarean section operation to facilitate delivery of the impacted head. Am J Obstet Gynaecol 1984; 148:707–710.
18. Lippert TH. Abdominovaginal delivery in case of impacted head in cesarean operation. Am J Obstet Gynecol 1985; 151:703.
19. Blickstein I. Difficult delivery of the impacted fetal head during cesarean section: intraoperative disengagement dystocia. J Perinat Med 2004; 32:465–469.
20. Berhan Y, Berhan A. A meta-analysis of reverse breech extraction to deliver a deeply impacted head during cesarean delivery. Int J Gynaecol Obstet 2014; 124:99–105.
21. Murless BG. Foetal head extractors and lower uterine section. BJOG 1954; 61:116–120.
22. Weisman AI, Carrabba SR. Experiences with the Murless Head Extractor in cesarean section JAMA 1952; 150:1209.
23. Cerda Castellanos JL, Zavala Martinez JE, Matuta Raffray MM, Sevilla Enriquez L. Evaluation of the Murless head extractor Gunecol Obstet Mexi 1992; 60:322–325.
24. Barrier BF, Allison JL, Andelin CO, Drobnis EZ. A simple device prevents hysterotomy extensions during cesarean delivery for failed second stage of labor. Gynecol Obstet Invest 2013; 76:90–94.
25. Seal SL, Dey A, Barman SC, Kamily G, Myukherji J. Does elevating the fetal head prior to delivery using a fetal pillow reduce maternal and fetal complications in a full dilatation caesarean section? A prospective study with historical controls. JOG 2014; 34:241–244.
26. Seal SL, Dey A, Barman SC, Kamilya G, Murherji J, Onwude JL. Randomized controlled trial of elevation of the fetal head with a fetal pillow during cesarean delivery at full cervical dilatation. Int J Gynecol Obstet 2016; 133:178–182.
27. Vousden N, Tydeman G, Briley A, Seed PT, Shennan AH. Assessment of a vaginal device for delivery of the impacted fetal head at caesarean section. Int J Gynecol Obstet 2017; 37:157–161.

# Chapter 3

# Midwifery-led care for women at all levels of risk

*Sally K Tracy*

## INTRODUCTION

The State of the World's Midwifery report [1] which was released in 2014 by the World Health Organization (WHO) claimed that given greater investment in midwifery education and training, midwives could reduce maternal and newborn deaths by two-thirds. Following the release of this report the Lancet published a series of international studies on midwifery outlining a framework for quality maternal and newborn care [2,3]. The unanimous recommendation was a shift from fragmented maternal and newborn care to a whole-system approach with midwifery as the key component to its success.

Although there is international agreement on the definition of the midwife adopted by the International Confederation of Midwives (ICM 2005) and endorsed by FIGO and the WHO, in many parts of the world there are considerable variations in the education and role of the midwife and the organisation and delivery of maternity services. For example, in New Zealand the midwife is the nominated 'lead maternity carer' regardless of place of birth [4]; in countries such as the Netherlands and Scandinavia and most of Europe and Australia care is offered primarily by midwives, whilst in the US and North America obstetrician led care is the norm.

The international definition of the midwife clearly states the necessary qualifications for midwifery practice, the types of care that can be given by midwives and the locations where midwives can practice.

> **Global definition of a midwife (ICM 2005)**
>
> A midwife is a person who, having been regularly admitted to a midwifery educational programme, duly recognised in the country in which it is located, has successfully completed the prescribed course of studies in midwifery and has acquired the requisite qualifications to be registered and/or legally licensed to practice midwifery. The midwife is recognised as a responsible and accountable professional who works in partnership with women to give the necessary support, care and advice during pregnancy, labour and the postpartum period, to conduct births on the midwife's own responsibility and to provide care for the

---

**Sally K Tracy** DMID MA BNURS RM RGON, Professor of Midwifery, University of Sydney; conjoint University of New South Wales, Sydney, Australia

> newborn and the infant. This care includes preventative measures, the promotion of normal birth, the detection of complications in mother and child, the accessing of medical care or other appropriate assistance and the carrying out of emergency measures. The midwife has an important task in health counselling and education, not only for the woman, but also within the family and the community. This work should involve antenatal education and preparation for parenthood and may extend to women's health, sexual or reproductive health and child care. A midwife may practice in any setting including the home, community, hospitals, clinics or health units.

In the following chapter, the term 'caseload midwifery care' is used interchangably with Midwifery Group Practice (MGP) and midwifery-led care. The aim of caseload midwifery is to provide women with the same midwife (or small group practice of midwives) to provide the full complement of midwifery care from booking in through until discharge from care at 4-6 weeks following the birth of the baby. In this way, care is centred completely on the woman and her family within an integrated, collaborative framework [5]. Evidence shows that continuity models have an impact on improving safety, clinical outcomes, as well as a better experience; and there appears to be a reduction in pre-term births through continuity of the care [6].

Following the introduction of 'Changing Childbirth' [7] in 1993, the first caseload practices were established in two London teaching hospitals to introduce the principles of choice, continuity and control for women [8]. From the start, caseload care was offered to women with no identified risk factors, however, this is dramatically changing with the realisation that collaboration and co-ordination of care with other health professionals does not detract from the practice of midwifery-led care when women are referred for expert care alongside the midwifery care they receive. With the move to caseload care in the UK, midwives experienced an enhanced sense of personal and professional autonomy [9]. They were able to take responsibility and make decisions and practice the 'full scope' of midwifery. Twenty years on from the 'Changing Childbirth' report Better Births – the National Maternity Review released by the NHS in 2016 promises to build on these achievements and promote further implementation of caseload care in the NHS [10].

## CHILDBIRTH TODAY AMIDST THE CASCADE OF INTERVENTIONS

Amongst the resource rich nations of the world pregnancy and childbirth are generally very safe for the majority of women and their babies. There is nevertheless growing concern at the increasing levels of obstetric intervention amongst childbearing women [11]. Rising intervention rates are most clearly reflected in the changes in rates of caesarean section (CS) that have been rising gradually for many years – from about 10% of births 30 years ago to near 25% of births in NHS hospitals in England in 2013–2014; and at similar rates of increase in European countries, Australia, Canada and the US. In 2013, CS rates were lowest in Nordic countries (Iceland, Finland, Sweden and Norway), Israel and the Netherlands [12]. Worldwide the prevalence of CS correlates with socioeconomic status so that in resource poor countries even medically indicated CS are rarely available. In contrast, lower-middle-income countries have some of the highest rates in the world, especially among the more affluent women who seek more 'medicalised' health care within private delivery systems [13]. In 2016, an ecological study compiling all available CS rates worldwide using country-level data from 159 countries and representing 98.0% of global live births in 2005 found no corresponding improvement in perinatal outcomes associated with CS rates when the CS rate exceeded 10% [14].

In addition to CS, linked population based data in Australia has revealed that amongst women with uncomplicated pregnancies, a third of all women currently have some form of intervention such as an induction or augmentation of their labour combined with an epidural [15] and that this trend shows no sign of decreasing [16]. Cost modelling of these interventions showed a relative cost increase of up to 50% for low risk primiparous women and up to 36% for low risk multiparous women as labour interventions accumulated [17].

Not only do interventions impact on the cost of services, they carry with them the potential for serious morbidities for mother and infant. Caesarean births carry the risk of morbidity associated with surgery [18] and possible maternal complications in subsequent pregnancies (e.g. uterine rupture, placenta praevia, and placenta accreta) [18–20]. Operative birth also increases the fetal risks of respiratory distress syndrome [21] persistent pulmonary hypertension [22] and admission to special care or neonatal intensive care (NICU) nurseries particularly if the CS is performed before the onset of labour [21,23–25]. Meta-analyses of cohort and case-control studies of CS reveal latent risks for chronic disease such as type 1 diabetes mellitus, [26] asthma, [27,28] and obesity [29].

The public health concern regarding the apparent inevitability of a rising caesarean rate [30] has resulted in policies designed to promote a lower rate of operative birth and increase the rate of normal vaginal birth. In the US, Healthy People 2020 set a national objective to reduce caesarean births among low risk first time mothers at full-term by 10% over the next 10 years [31]. Similar policies have been promoted in the UK [32]. In Australia most states and territories have introduced policy directives similar to the New South Wales 'Towards Normal Birth' policy directive aimed at explicitly, increasing the vaginal birth rate and decreasing the CS rate [33]. Many of these government policies recommend women having midwifery-led care in an effort to reduce the CS rate.

## DOES CONTINUITY OF MIDWIFERY CARE IMPROVE OUTCOMES?

In 2010, a UK-wide collaboration of the four UK Chief Nursing and Midwifery Officers in partnership with the Royal Colleges published a manifesto, Midwifery 2020 [34]. The aim was to consolidate the achievements that midwifery has made and to identify any changes needed to the way midwives work to fulfil women's health and social needs and expectations [34].

The report recommended that midwives take a lead professional role planning and providing a woman's care, with her input and agreement, from initial antenatal assessment through to the end of the postnatal period. In most circumstances, a midwife would take the role of lead professional for all healthy women with straightforward pregnancies.

In that same year, a clinical redesign of maternity services was undertaken at two tertiary teaching hospitals in Australia [35]. The aim was to move away from the current thinking that midwifery continuity of care could only be safely offered to low risk women and assess the clinical outcomes and cost of providing midwifery-led care for all women irrespective of risk factors compared to standard or routine hospital care through a randomised controlled trial (RCT), the M@NGO (Midwives at New Group Practice Options) trial [36].

It was hypothesised that a re-structure of the maternity service to provide midwifery continuity of care from the first hospital visit to postnatal discharge might reduce interventions in childbirth, reduce costs and increase women's satisfaction. The re-structure was called 'caseload midwifery' and aimed to dramatically reduce the fragmentation of care and the need to have multiple care providers. Unlike the earlier studies of midwifery-led models, this program was designed to offer midwife led care or caseload care to women regardless of medical, obstetric or social risk factors.

The differences between caseload and standard midwifery care are described in **Table 3.1**.

Standard or routine hospital care may involve shared care from a general practitioner or private obstetrician and hospital midwives. It is provided through antenatal clinics, labour wards, and postnatal wards, where care is provided by rostered medical and midwifery staff. In standard care, women might potentially see a different midwife for every visit. The majority of childbearing women in Australia receive this option of care based on a fragmented system where women meet multiple midwifery and obstetric staff at each consultation throughout the course of pregnancy, birth and the postnatal period. This is similar to findings in the UK where a study of 10,000 women in 2014 reported that very few labouring women had one midwife caring for them through labour (16%); a quarter (26%) had four or more midwives providing care; and a high proportion of women (85%) reported not having previously met any of the midwives caring for them during labour and birth [37].

## THE M@NGO TRIAL OF CASELOAD CARE FOR WOMEN IRRESPECTIVE OF RISK

At the outset, the M@NGO trial [36] entailed a clinical redesign of the maternity service to offer caseload care for a third of all women. The existing birth suite services were reconfigured to a single clinical unit, under a single birth services management structure. The changes resulted in the establishment of 12 Midwifery Group Practices (MGPs) made up of four full-time equivalent (FTE) midwives in each group undertaking caseload midwifery care [35]. In this model of caseload care for women of all risk the caseload midwife became the named midwife for 35–40 women each year and coordinated each woman's care in collaboration with the other members of her group practice. Each MGP was assigned a designated collaborating obstetrician who worked closely with two to three practice groups (usually about 8–12 midwives). Women had continuity of care and carer during pregnancy, birth and after birth from the named midwife or one of the other three midwives within the MGP. The collaborating obstetricians met at regular intervals with the midwives and were available for telephone communication or individual clinical consultation for women with increasing complexity. Clear plans of care, including referral to specialist services, were negotiated and documented with input from the women, the caseload midwife and the obstetrician.

An integral factor in this model was the strong collaborative relationship between the MGP midwives and their nominated consultant obstetrician. Referral to medical or other services occurred as necessary using the Australian National Midwifery Consultation and Referral Guidelines [38]. Weekly multi-disciplinary meetings that often involved peer review, with the specialist consultant for each group were necessary for maintaining skills and staff development. An evaluation of the dynamics of the professional relationships in this collaborative model of clinical consultation between the obstetrician and midwives was published in 2012 [39].

### Table 3.1 Factors that differentiate midwifery-led care (caseload care) and standard hospital care [36]

| | Midwife-led care (caseload care) | Standard or routine care |
|---|---|---|
| Annual salary versus Rostered shift work | Caseload midwives are employed on an annualised salary; they work in cycles of 152 hours over 4 weeks; and do not work in excess of 12 hours consecutively in any 24-hour period [40] | Rostered midwives are paid on the basis of their years of service and whether they are full time (38 hours per week) or part time; they are employed to provide a rostered service in 8 or 12 hours shifts |
| Self-managed time versus Rostered shifts | Caseload midwives potentially match workload to need; each midwife cares for about 40 women per annum; and provides back-up for an additional 40 women | Midwives are rostered prospectively; to match actual workload and number of midwives prospectively rostered on any ward for any given shift is not possible |
| Continuity of carer versus Fragmented care | Women receive continuity of care from a named midwife or her small group practice of midwives for the duration of pregnancy, labour, birth and postnatal care, ensuring consistency of advice and information | Routine care is offered by midwives working in designated separate ward or clinic areas; they do not have the opportunity to follow each woman through the duration of care |
| Named midwife versus Unknown carer | Having a known or named midwife encourages women to become active participants in decision making around pregnancy care | Women booked under team of the day might feel uninvolved in decision making; exposure to multiple carers might make women anxious about having to repeat information |
| Individual antenatal assessment versus Antenatal clinics | Antenatal assessments are tailored to the woman's needs in the community or home; combined antenatal/postnatal groups are possible | Women attend routine antenatal clinics in accordance with hospital policies; antenatal classes are offered in the hospital or community |
| Labour is assessed before admission versus Admit before assessment | Women phone their caseload midwife to discuss their progress of labour before being admitted to labour ward, thereby potentially avoiding unnecessary hours spent in hospital and increasing the possibility of interventions to accelerate progress | Women phone the labour ward before arriving at hospital at the onset of labour; they might not have previously met the midwife |
| Early discharge and home postnatal visits versus Hospital postnatal care | Women are encouraged to go home early and are visited by their caseload midwife at home in the first few hours after birth, then at home or in the community for up to 6 weeks or 10 visits | Women receive postnatal care in hospital; a domiciliary follow-up visit from a rostered community midwife might take place if the woman meets the criteria for early discharge – before 48 hours for vaginal birth and 72 hours for caesarean section |
| Consultation and referral | Collaboration between medical staff and caseload midwives is guided by the Australian National Midwifery Guidelines for Consultation and Referral [38] | Midwives have access to the Australian National Midwifery Guidelines for Consultation and Referral [38] |

Midwives offering caseload care are employed by the health service on an annualised salary agreement. This is the single most significant factor enabling the differentiation between the way midwives have traditionally provided care in hospitals compared with midwife led care described here. In 2008, in response to the need for a new industrial order for the emerging caseload midwifery models of care in Australia, most states initiated a new industrial award similar to that in New South Wales, the 'Model Pilot Agreement for Midwifery Caseload Practice Annualised Salary Agreement' [40].

To achieve a sustainable level of flexibility MGP midwives work within group practices of four midwives employed under these state approved industrial awards. Caseload midwives are employed within the public hospital system on an annualised salary comprising their base rate salary according to their years of experience and up to a 29% loading to compensate for penalty and on-call allowances. This is designed to give wage parity with other midwives working in hospitals on a rostered and rotating shift pattern. In Australia, the industrial awards differ slightly between states but in general the caseload midwife is required to work a cycle of 152 hours over a 4-week time period with a minimum of 9 and a maximum of 12 rostered days off. Australian industrial award agreements state that midwives should not work in excess of 12 consecutive hours in any 24-hour period [19]. These industrial constraints provide a framework for clinical safety and a buffer for professional burnout in addition to the flexibility that enables midwives to self-manage their workloads and respond directly to the needs of the women enrolled in their care. The provision of continuity of carer is difficult to achieve in maternity services in which most midwives have become accustomed to working shifts [41,42], however, the M@NGO trial found that midwives working within this industrial award were able to provide the large majority of women with their known caseload or backup caseload midwife in labour, compared with only a small proportion in the standard care group. During the study, 759 (87%) women in the caseload group had their known caseload midwife or their backup caseload midwife with them in labour, compared with only 123 (14%) women in the standard care group who had met their midwife before going into labour [36]. Each MGP is encouraged to design a work schedule that suits the members of the group according to family and other life commitments. These work plans have enabled midwives within group practices to maintain a healthy balance in their working lives while employed by the public hospital system and meeting the needs of individual woman in their group practice. A sustainable workforce model has evolved where MGP midwives may arrange their on call for alternate nights and weekends; or other configurations that are mutually agreed within the group practice [35].

In Australia, as in other resource rich nations childbirth accounts for the highest number of occupied bed days [43]; however, the current structure of public maternity systems makes it challenging to deliver value for money. Financing arrangements based on traditional long-standing approaches to public hospital funding directs maternity care into the acute care setting where specialist obstetric care is prioritised while limiting the role of midwives [43]. Maternity care is unique as the services support predominantly healthy women through a natural life event that does not always require a doctor-led intervention [37].

The evaluation of caseload care through the latest Cochrane systematic review suggests the future is very promising for midwife led care [6]. Fifteen trials (including the M@NGO trial) were included involving 17,674 women. For the primary outcomes, women who had midwife-led continuity models of care were less likely to experience regional analgesia [risk ratio (RR) 0.85, 95% confidence interval (CI) 0.78 to 0.92; participants = 17,674]; instrumental vaginal birth (RR 0.90, 95% CI 0.83 to 0.97; participants = 17,501; preterm birth <37 weeks (RR 0.76, 95% CI 0.64 to 0.91; participants = 13,238; all fetal loss before and after 24 weeks plus neonatal death (RR 0.84, 95% CI 0.71 to 0.99; participants = 17,561). Women who had midwife-led continuity models of care were more likely to experience spontaneous vaginal birth (RR 1.05, 95% CI 1.03 to 1.07; participants = 16,687).

There were no differences between groups for caesarean births or intact perineum. For the secondary outcomes, women who had midwife-led continuity models of care were less likely to experience amniotomy (RR 0.80, 95% CI 0.66 to 0.98; participants = 3,253; episiotomy) (average RR 0.84, 95% CI 0.77 to 0.92; participants = 17,674) and fetal loss less than 24 weeks and neonatal death (RR 0.81, 95% CI 0.67 to 0.98; participants = 15,645). Women who had midwife-led continuity models of care were more likely to experience no intrapartum analgesia or anaesthesia (RR 1.21, 95% CI 1.06 to 1.37; participants = 10,499) and more likely to be attended at birth by a known midwife (RR 7.04, 95% CI 4.48 to 11.08; participants = 6,917). There were no differences between groups for fetal loss equal to or after 24 weeks.

Results of the Australian M@NGO trial – which was the first RCT of midwife-led care for women irrespective of risk factors reflected many of these outcomes [36]. The study found a significantly lower rate of CS before the onset of labour (elective CS) [69 (8%) versus 94 (11%); OR 0.72, 95% CI 0.52–0.99; $P$ = 0.05]. This is significant given the mounting concern regarding the immunological and metabolic differences between infants born before the onset of labour and those who experience labour [44] and the evidence that women with a primary elective CS without labour are more likely, compared with those undergoing primary emergency CS with labour, to develop an accreta in a subsequent pregnancy with placenta praevia [45].

Although the predominant model of care worldwide continues to offer women very fragmented care in the hospital system, the M@NGO study found one-to-one midwifery care was safe for women irrespective of their risk status. The study found that with the right level of communication and collaboration with obstetricians and physicians [39], the midwifery-led component is quite safe to offer for women with pregnancies complicated with medical, obstetric and social risk factors [36].

Midwifery-led models of care are associated with an increased likelihood of maternal satisfaction across antenatal, intrapartum and postnatal care [46]. Caseload midwifery is a complex intervention because it has a number of interacting components that act both independently and interdependently. These complex networks can have powerful and pervasive effects on how systems actually perform and function [47,48] In the case of the caseload model described [36], performance and function are affected by factors such as enhanced senior management support, clear governance structures and communication, clinical engagement, and give and take between professionals [49]. In addition to this, one of the most compelling outcomes of the M@NGO trial was the reduction in overall CS rate from the base rate of 29% at the beginning of the trial to 22% in the standard group and 21% in the trial group [36]. This may have been due to the Hawthorn effect, however, given that more than one-third of women in the tertiary teaching hospital were receiving the intervention, the restructuring of midwifery care to caseload midwifery might have positively affected clinical practice in the standard care model, particularly within the birth environment. Nevertheless the decrease in CS represented more than a 25% reduction compared with Australian national rates in 2012. In the 6 years since the trial ended the CS rate has remained at 21–23% in the caseload groups whilst returning to 31% amongst those receiving standard care. In the caseload groups while those receiving the standard rostered care have a CS rate of 31% at present (Personal communication, Directors of Obstetric services, Royal Hospital for Women, Sydney.). Preliminary findings from the follow-up studies planned for long-term outcomes of midwife led care have shown some promising moderating effects on maternal stress during birth [50].

A cost reduction from a reorganisation of the way in which care is delivered in the public hospital system could play a major part in reducing public health expenditure. In the case of the M@NGO trial [36], small differences in most clinical outcome measures in favour of caseload midwifery accounted for the lower median cost for caseload midwifery than for standard care. In the caseload group higher proportions of women with spontaneous onset of labour, unassisted vaginal birth, using less pharmacological analgesia for labour; and fewer women having a postpartum blood loss >500 mL, combined with one fewer antenatal visit and a significant reduction in the postnatal stay in hospital in the caseload group led to a significant reduction in cost per woman for caseload midwifery. Amongst the neonates there were fewer babies admitted to the NICU from the caseload group. Given that one day in the neonatal care unit can cost in advance of $2,000 per day, fewer admissions amount to large savings. The two groups had similar outcomes in terms of the health of the mother and baby, however, women who were cared for by the same midwife throughout their pregnancy, labour and after birth saved the public health system around $566·74 less per woman; and a saving of $271.43 per infant.

## CONCLUSION

The recent maternity services review in England, Better Births [10], reported that women preferred to be cared for by one midwife or a small group of midwives. The report recommended that midwives who work in a continuity of care caseload group practice need their time to be 'ring-fenced', and not diverted to other services. This allows for flexible working where midwives manage their own diary, in conjunction with the rest of their colleagues.

The report also recommended that a scheme called the NHS Personal Maternity Care Budget aimed at providing a simple mechanism to enable women to make a choice in selecting their chosen accredited provider would be trialled in several areas within 2016-2017, supported by NHS England [10]. In New Zealand, a similar scheme has been working since 1990, giving women the choice of their lead maternity carer and a choice about place of birth [4]. The Independent Hospital Pricing Authority in Australia is currently also looking at the prospect of introducing a bundled maternity payment which would allow for district health boards to offer innovative maternity models, including more midwifery-led care. MGP models may play a major role in the future, reducing the public health burden by increasing normal outcomes and promoting more efficient use of funds.

Every year in England there are almost 700,000 live births. In 2012/13, the associated maternity care cost the NHS around £2.6 billion which is the equivalent to an average of £3,700 per birth [51].

Given the significant variation in safety, effectiveness and outcomes between providers that cannot be explained on the basis of differences in demography, deprivation or clinical complexity in many resource rich nations such as the UK [10], Europe [52], Australia [53] and the US [54] it is clearly time to look at new ways of offering maternity care.

The configuration of the caseload model differs substantially from standard midwifery care (**Table 3.1**). Caseload midwifery care appears to work in the maternity system by intercepting some of the pathways that can contribute to increased obstetric intervention. It works on the assumption that women will labour more effectively, need to stay in hospital less time, and feel a stronger sense of satisfaction and personal control if they have the opportunity to get to know their midwife in a partnership relationship [55,56] rather than rely on unfamiliar hospital staff during their pregnancy and maternity care.

Evidence shows that continuity models have an impact on improving safety, reducing preterm birth and providing a better experience for women [6]. There is also compelling evidence that women with identified risk factors during pregnancy and birth have improved outcomes where their care is co-ordinated as required between midwifery, specialist and obstetric services under a midwifery-led model of midwifery care regardless of risk.

> **Key points for clinical practice**
> - Caseload midwifery models of care for all women regardless of risk have been established in a variety of community based and hospital settings. They report a reduction in clinical intervention rates while maintaining the safety of mothers and babies through effective interdisciplinary collaboration and consultation.
> - Caseload midwifery care appears to work in the maternity system by intercepting some of the pathways contributing to medical intervention. Women labour more effectively, need to stay in hospital less time, and feel a stronger sense of satisfaction and personal control if they have the opportunity to get to know their midwife in a partnership relationship rather than rely on unfamiliar hospital staff during their pregnancy and maternity care.
> - Successful caseload midwifery practice requires midwives to be contracted or employed on an annualised salary that supports a high level of self-management. This will ensure midwives are available to respond to the needs of women who are booked with them as the named midwife.
> - Implementing caseload midwifery through MGPs within the mainstream maternity services has far reaching implications for the retention and recruitment of midwives.
> - Strategies used to achieve a large sustainable clinical service redesign introducing caseload midwifery require factors such as enhanced senior management support, clear governance structures and communication, clinical engagement, and give and take between professionals.
> - MGP models may play a major role in the future, reducing the public health burden by increasing normal outcomes and promoting more efficient use of funds.

## REFERENCES

1. UNFPA, ICM, WHO. The State of the World's Midwifery 2014. A Universal Pathway . A Women's Right to Health. 2014.
2. Homer CS, Friberg IK, Dias MA, et al. The projected effect of scaling up midwifery. The Lancet 2014; 384:1146–1157.
3. ten Hoope-Bender P, de BL, Campbell J, et al. Improvement of maternal and newborn health through midwifery. The Lancet 2014; 384:1226–1235.
4. Grigg CP, Tracy SK. New Zealand's unique maternity system. Women and Birth 2013; 26:59–64.
5. Tracy SK, Hartz D, Nicholl M, McCann Y, Latta D. An integrated service network in maternity – the implementation of a midwifery-led unit. Aust Health Rev 2005; 29:332–339.
6. Sandall J, Soltani H, Gates S, Shennan A, Devane D. Midwife-led continuity models versus other models of care for childbearing women. Cochrane Database Syst Rev 2016; 4:CD004667.
7. Department of Health. Changing Childbirth: the Report of the Expert Maternity Group. HMSO.London, 1993.
8. McCourt C, Page L. Report on the evaluation of One-to-One midwifery. London: Thames Valley University, 1996.
9. Sandall J. Occupational burnout in midwives: new ways of working and the relationship between organisational factors and psychological health and wellbeing. Risk, Decision & Policy 1998; 3:213–232.

10. NHS. BETTER BIRTHS: Improving outcomes of maternity services in England. London UK: NHS; 2016.
11. MacLennan A, Nelson KB, Hankins G, Speer M. Who Will Deliver Our Grandchildren? Implications of Cerebral Palsy Litigation. JAMA 2005; 249:1688–1690.
12. OECD. Health at a Glance 2015. Paris: OECD; 2015.
13. Betran AP, Ye J, Moller AB, et al. The Increasing Trend in Caesarean Section Rates: Global, Regional and National Estimates: 1990-2014. PLoS One 2016; 11:e0148343.
14. Ye J, Zhang J, Mikolajczyk R, Torloni MR, Gulmezoglu AM, Betran AP. Association between rates of caesarean section and maternal and neonatal mortality in the 21st century: a worldwide population-based ecological study with longitudinal data. BJOG 2016; 123:745–753.
15. Tracy SK, Sullivan E, Wang YA, Black D, Tracy M. Birth outcomes associated with interventions in labour amongst low risk women: a population-based study. Women and Birth 2007; 20:41–48.
16. Dahlen HG, Tracy S, Tracy M, Bisits A, Brown C, Thornton C. Rates of obstetric intervention among low-risk women giving birth in private and public hospitals in NSW: a population-based descriptive study. BMJ Open 2014; 2.
17. Tracy SK, Tracy MB. Costing the cascade: estimating the cost of increased obstetric intervention in childbirth using population data. BJOG 2003; 110:717–724.
18. Lydon-Rochelle M, Holt VL, Martin DP, Easterling TR. Association between method of delivery and maternal rehospitalization. JAMA 2000; 283:2411–2416.
19. Green L, Knight M, Seeney FM, et al. The epidemiology and outcomes of women with postpartum haemorrhage requiring massive transfusion with eight or more units of red cells: a national cross-sectional study. BJOG 2016; 123:2164–2170.
20. Lydon-Rochelle M, Holt VL, Easterling TR, Martin DP. First-birth cesarean and placental abruption or previa at second birth(1). Obstet Gynecol 2001; 97:765–769.
21. Morrison JJ, Rennie JM, Milton PJ. Neonatal respiratory morbidity and mode of delivery at term: influence of timing of elective caesarean section. BJOG 1995; 102:101–106.
22. Jain L, Dudell GG. Respiratory transition in infants delivered by cesarean section. Semin Perinatol 2006; 30:296–304.
23. Kolas T, Saugstad OD, Daltveit AK, Nilsen ST, Oian P. Planned cesarean versus planned vaginal delivery at term: comparison of newborn infant outcomes. Am J Obstet Gynecol 2006; 195:1538–1543.
24. Tracy SK, Tracy MB, Sullivan E. Admission of term infants to neonatal intensive care: a population-based study. Birth 2007; 34:301–307.
25. Kupari M, Talola N, Luukkaala T, Tihtonen K. Does an increased cesarean section rate improve neonatal outcome in term pregnancies? Arch Gynecol Obstet 2016; 294:41–46.
26. Cardwell CR, Stene LC, Joner G, et al. Caesarean section is associated with an increased risk of childhood-onset type 1 diabetes mellitus: a meta-analysis of observational studies. Diabetologia 2008; 51:726–735.
27. Black M, Bhattacharya S, Philip S, Norman JE, McLernon DJ. Planned Cesarean Delivery at Term and Adverse Outcomes in Childhood Health. JAMA 2015; 314:2271–2279.
28. Thavagnanam S, Fleming J, Bromley A, Shields MD, Cardwell CR. A meta-analysis of the association between Caesarean section and childhood asthma. Clin Exp Allergy 2008; 38:629–633.
29. Li HT, Zhou YB, Liu JM. The impact of cesarean section on offspring overweight and obesity: a systematic review and meta-analysis. Int J Obes (Lond) 2013; 37:893–899.
30. Declercq E, Young R, Cabral H, Ecker J. Is a Rising Cesarean Delivery Rate Inevitable? Trends in Industrialized Countries, 1987 to 2007. Birth 2011; 38:99–104.
31. US Department of Health and Human Services. Healthy People 2020. Washington DC, US Department of Health and Human Services, 2010.
32. Strategic Clinical Networks London N. London Maternity Strategic Clinical Network (2015) Increasing the number of women who receive continuity of midwife care: A best practice toolkit NHS London. London, NHS UK, 2015.
33. New South Wales Health. Maternity – Towards Normal Birth in NSW PD2010_045. Sydney, Australia: NSW Health; 2011.
34. DOH. Midwifery 2020: Delivering expectations. London, UK: DOH; 2010.
35. Hartz DL, White J, Lainchbury KA, et al. Australian maternity reform through clinical redesign. Australian Health Review 2012; 36:169–175.
36. Tracy SK, Hartz DL, Tracy MB, Allen J, Forti A, Hall B, et al. Caseload midwifery care versus standard maternity care for women of any risk: M@NGO, a randomised controlled trial. The Lancet 2013; 382:1723–1732.

37. Redshaw M, Henderson J. Safely Delivered: a national survey of women's experience of maternity care, 2014. Oxford UK: National Perinatal Epidemiology Unit; 2015.
38. Australian College of Midwives. National Midwifery Guidelines for Referral and Consultation (3rd Edition), 2013.
39. Beasley S, Ford N, Tracy SK, Welsh AW. Collaboration in Maternity Care is achievable and practical. Aust N Z J Obstet Gynaecol 2012; 52:576–581.
40. NSW Department of Health and NSW Nurses' Association. Model Pilot Agreement for Midwifery Caseload Practice Annualised Salary Agreement. Policy Document Number IB2008_012 2011. Ministry of Health NSW Pilot Model Annualised Salary Agreement for Midwifery Group Practices 2014 https://www1.health.nsw.gov.au/pds/ActivePDSDocuments/IB2014_050.pdf
41. Finlay S, Sandall J. "Someone's rooting for you": continuity, advocacy and street-level bureaucracy in UK maternal healthcare. Soc Sci Med 2009; 69:1228–1235.
42. Page L, McCourt C, Beake S, Vail A, Hewison J. Clinical interventions and outcomes of One-to-One midwifery practice. J Public Health Med 1999; 21:243–248.
43. Commonwealth of Australia . Report of the Maternity Services Review 2009 http://www.health.gov.au/internet/main/publishing.nsf/Content/maternityservicesreview-report Accessed. http://www.health.gov.au/internet/main/publishing.nsf/Content/maternityservicesreview-report
44. Sinha A, Bewley S, McIntosh T. Myth: babies would choose prelabour caesarean section. Semin Fetal Neonatal Med 2011; 16:247–253.
45. Kamara M, Henderson JJ, Doherty DA, Dickinson JE, Pennell CE. The risk of placenta accreta following primary elective caesarean delivery: a case-control study. BJOG 2013; 120:879–886.
46. McLachlan HL, Forster DA, Davey MA, et al. The effect of primary midwife-led care on women's experience of childbirth: results from the COSMOS randomised controlled trial. BJOG 2016; 123:465–474.
47. Braithwaite J, Runciman WB, Merry AF. Towards safer, better healthcare: harnessing the natural properties of complex sociotechnical systems. Qual Saf Health Care 2009; 18:37–41.
48. UK MRC. Developing and evaluating complex interventions: new guidance. London UK: Medical Research Council; 2008.
49. Macfarlane F, Greenhalgh T, Humphrey C, et al. A new workforce in the making? A case study of strategic human resource management in a whole-system change effort in healthcare. J Health Organ Manag 2011; 25:55–72.
50. King S, Kildea S, Austin MP, et al. QF2011: a protocol to study the effects of the Queensland flood on pregnant women, their pregnancies, and their children's early development. BMC Pregnancy Childbirth 2015; 15:109.
51. National Audit Office Department of Health. Maternity services in England, 2013.
52. Macfarlane AJ, Blondel B, Mohangoo AD, et al. Wide differences in mode of delivery within Europe: risk-stratified analyses of aggregated routine data from the Euro-Peristat study. BJOG 2016; 123:559–568.
53. Lee Yeun Yi, Roberts CL, Patterson JA, et al. Unexplained variation in hospital caesarean section rates. Medical Journal of Australia 2013; 199:348–353.
54. Kozhimannil KB, Law MR, Virnig BA. Cesarean delivery rates vary tenfold among US hospitals; reducing variation may address quality and cost issues. Health Aff (Millwood ) 2013; 32:527–535.
55. Guilliland K, Pairman S. The Midwifery Partnership: A model for practice. Victoria University of Wellington, NZ. Department of Nursing and Midwifery Monograph Series 95/1, 1995.
56. Page L. The New Midwifery. Churchill Livingstone. London; 2000.

# Chapter 4

# The role of urodynamics in female lower urinary tract symptoms

*Verghese TS, Latthe P*

## INTRODUCTION

Lower urinary tract dysfunction produces a huge burden on sufferers in particular and on society in general. Urinary incontinence (UI) can adversely affect the physical, psychological and social well being of the affected individual, as well their friends and family [1]. There are also significant financial implications, which include the costs of pads, prescription costs and time off work [2].

In a population based cross-sectional survey in five European countries, out of a total of 19,165 individuals, 64.3% reported at least one of the lower urinary tract symptoms (LUTS). Nocturia was the most prevalent LUTS (men, 48.6%; women, 54.5%). The prevalence of storage LUTS (men, 51.3%; women, 59.2%) was greater than that for voiding (men, 25.7%; women, 19.5%) and post micturition (men, 16.9%; women, 14.2%) symptoms combined. The overall prevalence of overactive bladder (OAB) was 11.8%; rates were similar in men and women and increased with age. OAB was more prevalent than all types of UI combined (9.4%) [1].

## LOWER URINARY TRACT

The lower urinary tract comprises of the bladder and urethra, which serves as a functional unit in the storage and voiding phase of the micturition cycle. The pelvic floor supports these two structures. LUTS are divided into storage, sensation, voiding and post-micturition symptoms [3] (**Table 4.1**). These symptoms can vary in severity and be present in different permutations and combinations.

The LUTS may be related to a variety of pathophysiological processes and assessment on the basis of symptoms alone can sometimes lead to an incorrect diagnosis, especially in patients with a neurogenic bladder. The need to support the clinical assessment with objective measurement has become accepted by most clinicians specialising in the care of patients with LUTS. Bladder diaries are useful in the investigation of LUTS and also to assess treatment response [4]. Completion of bladder diaries allows evaluation of fluid intake, fluid output and volumes voided as well as number of incontinence episodes and provoking factors. Urine dipstick, disease specific quality of life (QoL) questionnaires

---

**Verghese TS** MBBS, Clinical Research Fellow, Birmingham Woman's Hospital, Birmingham, UK

**Latthe P** MD, MRCOG, Consultant in Obstetrics and Gynaecology and Subspecialist in Urogynaecology, Birmingham Women's Hospital, Birmingham, UK

### Table 4.1 Symptoms of lower urinary tract

| Storage | Sensory | Voiding | Post-micturition |
|---|---|---|---|
| Frequency | Increased bladder sensation | Poor flow | Needing to revisit the toilet soon after voiding |
| Urgency | Reduced bladder sensation | Hesitancy | Post-voiding dribble |
| Nocturia | Absent bladder sensation | Intermittent flow | Feeling of incomplete emptying of bladder |
| Urinary incontinence | | Straining | – |
| – | | Terminal dribble | – |
| | | Spraying | |

and urodynamics are investigations that are used in evaluation of patients with LUTS. Uroflowmetry and measurement of post-void residual (PVR) urine by ultrasonography are noninvasive tests that can be routinely performed in patients with LUTS.

# URODYNAMICS

Multichannel urodynamics study (UDS) is a diagnostic assessment of the lower urinary tract. UDS is often described as the 'gold standard' for evaluating LUTS [5] as it is believed to reproduce the patient's symptoms to provide an explanation to the pathology.

It comprises of a series of interactive tests that look at the function of the bladder and urethra during both the filling and voiding phase.

The UDS consists of uroflowmetry, filling cystometry and pressure flow or voiding cystometry [6]. Uroflowmetry measures the flow rate during the voiding stage whilst multichannel cystometry evaluates the pressure and volume relationship in the bladder at both the filling and voiding stages.

Uroflowmetry is a noninvasive study of pattern of urine flow and the rate of voiding. It is performed by asking the patient with a comfortably full bladder to void in a flowmeter in privacy. Uroflowmetry is used to diagnose bladder outflow obstruction and also as a measure of detrusor contractility [7]. Filling cystometry is an invasive study of the storage function of the bladder. The variation in bladder pressure with incremental filling is graphically recorded as a cystometrogram. Detrusor pressure is recorded by subtracting abdominal pressure from the intravesical pressure. The rate of filling the bladder is generally between 30–100 mL/min depending on patient symptoms and is carried out interactively. Bladder sensation (first, normal and strong desire to void), bladder pain, detrusor activity, compliance of the bladder wall, incontinence and cystometric capacity is studied during the filling cystometry [8].

Voiding cystometry is the pressure volume relationship of the bladder during micturition. It begins when the 'instruction to void' is given by the urodynamicist and ends when the woman considers her voiding has finished. Measurements to be recorded should be the intravesical, intra-abdominal and detrusor pressures and the urine flow rate [9].

Universal antibiotic prophylaxis around urodynamics is not recommended. Prophylactic antibiotics do reduce the risk of bacteriuria after UDSs but there is not enough evidence to suggest that this reduced symptomatic urinary tract infections (UTIs) [10]. Patients who might benefit from periprocedure antibiotic prophylaxis are those with known relevant neurogenic lower urinary tract dysfunction, elevated PVRs, asymptomatic bacteriuria, immunosuppression, age over 70 years, and patients with any indwelling catheter or performing intermittent catheterisation [11].

Some studies have shown that UDS can be inaccurate and does not always correlate to the patient's symptoms [12-14]. There is no role for urodynamics prior to conservative management. The National Institute for Health and Care Excellence (NICE) states clearly that clinician should not perform multichannel cystometry, ambulatory urodynamics or videourodynamics before starting conservative management [15].

Multichannel urodynamics have poor sensitivity (50–80% false negative) for detrusor overactivity (DO) [16]. The bladder has been described as an unreliable witness because of the poor reproducibility of symptoms during UDSs. In a study on women with symptoms suggestive of pure stress incontinence, DO was found in 25% of the cases on urodynamics [17]. Ambulatory urodynamics is considered if the diagnosis is unclear after conventional urodynamics. Ambulatory urodynamics may have a higher pickup rate of DO and better correlation to clinical symptoms [18]. Literature reporting on ambulatory urodynamics is limited; it does appear to outperform conventional urodynamics in reaching a diagnosis. But its technical difficulty can affect results [19]. Objective data provided from the procedure may guide medical and surgical treatment [20].

There are two aims of the UDS test; these are to reproduce the patient's symptoms and secondly to provide a pathophysiological explanation for the patient's symptoms [21]. The International Urogynaecological Association (IUGA)/International Continence Society (ICS) joint report state and define the common diagnoses obtained following UDS which include DO, urodynamic stress incontinence (USI) and voiding dysfunction (VD). The report emphasises the need to correlate the sign, symptoms and urodynamic investigations in order to diagnose a condition [9].

## INDICATIONS

After undertaking a detailed clinical history, examination and conservative treatments, NICE recommends performing multichannel filling and voiding cystometry before surgery in women who have [15]:
- Symptoms of overactive bladder (OAB) leading to a clinical suspicion of DO
- Symptoms suggestive of VD or anterior compartment prolapse
- Previous surgery for stress incontinence

The NICE also recommends that the clinicians should offer video-urodynamic investigations to people who are known to have a high risk of renal complications (e.g. people with spina bifida, spinal cord injury or anorectal abnormalities). It recommends that clinicians offer UDS before performing surgical treatments for neurogenic lower urinary tract dysfunction [22].

The support for routine urodynamic testing in the management of women with UI or pelvic organ prolapse (POP) is eroding. The reasons for this change largely reflect the growing evidence that urodynamic testing in this context renders little additional information over basic office assessment [23].

## OVERACTIVE BLADDER

The OAB syndrome is a symptom complex of urinary urgency, usually accompanied by frequency and nocturia, with or without urgency urinary incontinence (UUI), in the absence of UTI or any proven pathology [9]. DO is the urodynamic observation characterised by the occurrence of involuntary detrusor contractions observed during the filling stage of UDS. These contractions can be spontaneous or provoked and may vary in duration and amplitude [9].

The pathology behind OAB symptoms may be DO in 54–58% of patients. A proportion of women, who have OAB symptoms, do not have a clinical diagnosis of DO following UDS [7]. One reason for this may be because UDS does not mimic the 'normal physiology' of the bladder. In a study of 2,737 women with UI symptoms, 1,626 (59%) reported mixed UI. Of these 42% had USI, 25% had pure DO, 18% had both DO and USI and 15% had normal UDS. In those with stress-predominant MUI, 64% had pure USI and in those with urgency-predominant MUI, only 47% had solely DO [24].

Patients with refractory OAB pose a therapeutic challenge. Approximately 25–40% of patients fail to achieve satisfactory improvement in incontinence with anticholinergics [25]. A multidisciplinary team review should be carried out before invasive therapy for UI. Guidelines such as those from the NICE recommend invasive treatments such as Botulinum toxin-A ((BTX-A), sacral neural stimulation (SNS), etc. only if there is DO on urodynamics [15]. A systematic review suggested that the outcomes in patients without ($n = 77$) or with ($n = 135$) DO were similar in the context of urodynamic findings, bladder diaries, QoL questionnaires, etc. when treated with BTX-A [odds ratio (OR) 1.52, 95% confidence interval (CI) 0.40 to 5.77] or SNS (OR 1.37, CI 0.76 to 2.48). The limited evidence suggests that urodynamic diagnosis of DO does not alter patient reported outcomes for invasive treatments such as BTX-A and SNS [26].

A prospective, longitudinal observational study, which was a part of the diagnostic accuracy of bladder ultrasound study (BUS), found that UDS appears to influence treatment decisions made by clinicians in determining treatment pathways in women presenting with OAB. Women treated based on UDS diagnoses appear to have greater reductions in symptoms than those who do not [27]. In a prospective questionnaire-based study, clinicians completed a pre- and post-UDS questionnaire on each UDS that they ordered. Overall, they felt that UDS was a clinically useful tool that altered the clinical impression and treatment plan in a large percentage of carefully selected patients [28].

The role of invasive urodynamics in the assessment of women with refractory overactive bladder symptoms is currently unclear. In an attempt to answer this important question the FUTURE (Female Urgency, Trial of Urodynamics as Routine Evaluation) randomised controlled trial (RCT) has been funded by the NIHR in the UK [29] to evaluate the clinical and cost effectiveness of invasive urodynamics over and above comprehensive clinical noninvasive assessment.

## STRESS URINARY INCONTINENCE

A recent meta-analysis of three studies where the women with stress urinary incontinence (SUI) or stress predominant mixed urinary incontinence (MUI) were randomised to either office evaluation ($n = 387$) or office evaluation and UDS ($n = 388$) found that was no statistical difference in the subjective outcome of success in the two groups [risk ratio 1.02 (95% CI 0.90–1.15)] or indeed in the rates of postoperative VD or urgency.

In women undergoing primary surgery for SUI or stress-predominant MUI without voiding difficulties, urodynamics does not improve outcomes – as long as the women undergo careful office evaluation [30].

The NICE also recommends that clinicians do not perform multichannel filling and voiding cystometry in women where pure SUI is diagnosed based on a detailed clinical history and examination [15].

Some clinicians routinely perform tests such as leak point pressures, urethral pressure profiles etc. Tests to differentiate between intrinsic sphincter deficiency (ISD) and urethral hypermobility are not recommended because of poor validity and reproducibility [31]. The retropubic midurethral sling works quite well as a first procedure for all types of SUI including urethral hypermobility and ISD [32].

## PROLAPSE

The role of UDSs before prolapse surgery is contentious. Previous studies in women with prolapse and women with uncomplicated SUI have focused on women without preoperative incontinence. Currently, it has not been possible to reach a universal consensus on the role of UDS before prolapse surgery in women with concomitant symptomatic or occult SUI.

Approximately quarter of continent women with POP develop UI post prolapse repair procedures [33]. The outcomes following vaginal prolapse repair and mid urethral sling (OPUS) trial demonstrated that concomitant continence surgery reduces the risk of postoperative iatrogenic SUI in women without SUI who are undergoing POP surgery. However, the trial also showed that combination surgery was associated with increased rates of complication such as bleeding, bladder perforation, prolonged catheterisation and UTIs [34]. Therefore, careful patient selection is extremely essential.

The effectiveness and safety of prolapse surgery versus combined prolapse and incontinence sling surgery in women with POP was studied in a systematic review which concluded that combination surgery reduces the risk of postoperative SUI, but short-term voiding difficulties and adverse events were more frequent after combination surgery [35] In a RCT, 134 women with symptomatic stage two or greater POP, and subjective or objective SUI without prolapse reduction, were randomised to prolapse repair with or without MUS. Women with prolapse and co-existing SUI were found to be less likely to suffer with SUI after transvaginal prolapse repair with MUS compared with prolapse repair only. However, only 17% of the women undergoing POP surgery needed additional mid urethral sling (MUS). A well-informed decision balancing risks and benefits of both strategies should be tailored to individual women [35]. Another systematic review concluded that prophylactic treatment of women with severe POP using retropubic midurethral sling was the only procedure that reduced the risk of UI [36].

Preoperative UDS with reduction of prolapse can help tailor the decision whether to perform concomitant continence operation as studies have shown negative predictive values for postoperative SUI of >90% [37]. Women with POP diagnosed with USI and normal bladder compliance with no DO are good candidates for combination prolapse and continence surgery such as retropubic tape. Insertion of a sling in women with occult SUI at the time of prolapse should be done based on shared decision-making between clinician and patient.

Preoperative UDS may also identify women at risk of persistent urgency, urgency incontinence and VD after POP surgery. The presence of preoperative DO and high voiding pressure at maximal flow along with higher bladder outlet obstruction index are predictive factors for complications postoperatively [38]. Identifying these patients allows clinicians to counsel and shape patient expectations as well as offer teaching intermittent selfcatheterisation. However, Nguyen et al. found that in approximately 75% of women with POP and symptomatic DO there is resolution of DO after prolapse repair [39] which can be one of the factors helpful to aid decision-making for women thinking about having prolapse surgery.

A retrospective study found that the incidence of de novo SUI after surgery for POP without occult SUI was 9.9% and was 4.4% in those without baseline complaint of SUI. Preoperatively, all patients had a negative stress test and no evidence of occult SUI on prolapse reduction during urodynamics. The patient can be counselled about the risk of de novo SUI and a staged procedure can be offered [40].

Prior to vaginal surgery, an individualised risk calculator may be used to inform presurgical counselling. In practice, many women are able to make this decision without specific numeric advice regarding individualised risk. In summary, there is no clear data to show that prior UDS can improve subjective or objective outcomes for prolapse. Current evidence on the role of UDS in women with POP is only to facilitate counselling of women undergoing surgery [41]. New well-designed randomised studies and cost analyses are necessary [42].

## VOIDING DIFFICULTIES/DYSFUNCTION

The true incidence of VD is unknown due to under diagnosis, variations in definition and under-reporting. Haylen et al. defined VD as a diagnosis by symptoms and urodynamic investigations, which are defined as abnormally slow and/or incomplete micturition [9].

Uroflowmetry assists in detecting abnormally slow flow rate and p PVR measurement detects high residual volumes. The diagnosis is based on repeated measurement to detect an abnormality. Pressure flow studies are indicated to evaluate the cause of any VD. This technique may assist in determining the nature of urethral obstruction. During normal urethral function, the urethra is open and continuously relaxed to allow micturition at a normal pressure, urine flow and PVR. However, in presence of reduced urine flow rate, raised PVR and increased detrusor pressure and flow rate, VD is diagnosed.

Surgery for SUI can be related to various degrees of outlet obstruction, de novo development of DO or worsening of pre-existing DO. The clinical challenge is to determine whether VD symptoms may be directly correlated to the outlet obstruction secondary to either tight sling placement or overzealous tightening of suspension sutures. The level of work up performed on these women would depend on the patient's level of 'bother' and willingness to risk possible intervention. Depending on the clinical situation, UDS is beneficial in documenting iatrogenic outlet obstruction as the cause for patient's symptoms.

Clinical symptom complex known as underactive bladder (UAB) is slowly gaining recognition. An UAB is defined as detrusor contractions with decreased strength resulting in slow stream and incomplete emptying of the bladder. This feature is identified in 12–45% of elderly population. The condition may arise due to myogenic failure or neuron signaling disruption. Currently there is lack of consensus regarding the urodynamic definition of UAB. In specific situations, invasive urodynamics may be helpful to distinguish bladder outlet obstruction from detrusor underactivity, although this distinction can be difficult. A common strategy is to measure contractility involves relating Pdet to urinary flow [43].

## QUALITY ASSURANCE

A key aspect of maintaining the accuracy of UDS is to ensure that the initial resting pressures are correct [44]. Previous studies have shown that reliability parameters can be poor despite standardised test-retest situations [45]. UDS can be further compromised by inconsistencies in clinical practices. Variations in the UDS procedure may vary from site to site and may be dependent upon the equipment and experience/training of the staff. Consistency and quality control is therefore paramount in UDS testing, particularly as the diagnoses/results may inform management decisions including invasive treatments such as surgery [5].

The need for standardisation in UDS is important if results are to be of high quality and reliable. There may be barriers to achieving standardisation in UDS due to infrastructure, staff attitudes and experience in performing UDS. In order to maintain reliability of urodynamic data, there should be standardisation of urodynamic technique, interpretation and performance [45].

## DRAWBACKS

Fear of pain refers to trait-like fear responses to painful situations, is a key component in medical fears [46] and may also influence willingness for invasive testing and follow-ups [47]. In one study, the perceived level of pain was strongly correlated with the level of apprehension and embarrassment during different steps of urodynamics. Younger age and apprehension were found to be significant risk factors for the heightened perception of pain on multivariate linear regression analyses [48]. The cross-sectional test accuracy study (BUS study) assessed the acceptability of UDS from the 687 participants [49]. Acceptability was evaluated in terms of pain and anxiety by completing Visual Analogue scores [50] and State- Trait Anxiety Inventory six-item short form (STAI-6) [51]. The response rates were 94% (646/687) and 87% (602/687) to the pain and anxiety questionnaire respectively [49]. The UDS procedure had statistically significant higher levels of pain and a lower rate of acceptability when compared to the bladder ultrasound procedure in detecting DO. In spite of these finding, the majority of the women were willing to have repeat UDS if needed in order to obtain a diagnosis or explanation for their bladder symptoms [49].

One of the important risks of UDS is that of developing UTI post procedure, 8% of women can develop a symptomatic UTI within 1 week of diagnosis of asymptomatic bacteruria. Every unit performing UDS should periodically audit their UTI rates following procedure and in addition have antibiotic treatment policies in place if the rates are higher than 5% [52].

The UDS is an interactive investigation that measures lower urinary tract function during urine storage and emptying. For most clinicians, common uncertainties include questions as to the optimal clinical conditions to perform urodynamic testing. The lack of reproducibility of UDS testing is another drawback centers encounter. This generally stems from physiological fluctuation in bladder function and also the inherent relative insensitivity in the instrument performing the tests [53].

## ALTERNATIVES TO URODYNAMICS

Bladder diaries are useful in the investigation of lower urinary tract symptoms (LUTS) and also to assess treatment response [4]. Completion of bladder diaries allows evaluation of fluid intake, fluid output and volumes voided as well as number of incontinence episodes and provoking factors.

The electronic Personal Assessment Questionnaire-Pelvic Floor (ePAQ-PF) is a computer-based tool to measure the impact of pelvic floor dysfunction on the women's QoL. The tool comprises of four domains – urinary, bowel, sexual and vaginal symptoms. McCooty et al. performed a prospective cohort study to identify the predictive value of ePAQ-PF in determining urodynamic diagnoses. The study recruited 390 women from a tertiary urogynaecology unit. OAB and SUI scores on the ePAQ-PF demonstrated that they are fair predictors in diagnosing DO and USI. As the OAB and SUI score on ePAQ-PF increased so did the likelihood of DO (up to a score of 75) and USI on UDS [54].

A prediction model called King's DO Score (KiDOS) has recently been developed. This prediction model comprises of six variables, which are established with history taking (parity, previous continence surgery), completion of validated symptom questionnaires and bladder diary. The factors considered the best predictors of DO were urgency UI, urge rating/ void and parity ($p < 0.01$). In addition the absence of SUI, vaginal bulging and previous continence surgery were also good predictors of DO ($P < 0.01$) [55].

A cross-sectional test accuracy study was undertaken to assess the accuracy of bladder wall thickness (BWT) in diagnosing DO in women with OAB symptoms There was no evidence that transvaginal BWT had any relationship with DO. Furthermore, BWT had no relationship to symptoms as measured by ICIQ-OAB score either on presentation or in the long term. BWT thus has no predictive or prognostic value as a test in this condition [49].

## SUMMARY

Urodynamic testing did change clinical decision-making in women treated for UI (RR 5.07, 95% CI 1.87 to 13.74) [56]. It seems intuitive that if clinicians have more information available to counsel their patients, care and outcomes should be improved. However, there is no evidence that the extra information provided by the investigation translates into better outcomes.

> **Key points for clinical practice**
> - There is no role for urodynamics prior to conservative management.
> - The NICE recommends performing UDS before surgery in women who have symptoms of OAB leading to a clinical suspicion of DO, VD or anterior prolapse and previous surgery for SUI.
> - The NICE encourages clinicians to offer UDS before performing surgical treatments for neurogenic lower urinary tract dysfunction
> - Urodynamics does not improve outcomes in women undergoing primary surgery for SUI or stress-predominant MUI without voiding difficulties, as long as thorough office evaluation is performed.
> - At present, the role of UDS in women with POP is only to facilitate counselling of women undergoing surgery but might not be cost effective.
> - Insertion of a sling in women with occult SUI at the time of prolapse repair should be subject to shared decision-making between clinician and patient.
> - UDS is beneficial in documenting iatrogenic outlet obstruction as the cause for patient's symptoms.
> - Robustly conducted randomised study data is needed to support the limited evidence suggesting that urodynamic diagnosis of DO does not alter patient reported outcomes for invasive treatments such as Botulinum toxin A cystoscopic injections or sacral neuromodulation.

# REFERENCES

1. Irwin DE, Milsom I, Hunskaar S, et al. Population-based survey of urinary incontinence, overactive bladder, and other lower urinary tract symptoms in five countries: results of the EPIC study. Eur Urol 2006; 50:1306–1314.
2. Irwin DE, Mungapen L, Milsom I, et al. The economic impact of overactive bladder syndrome in six Western countries. BJU Int 2009; 103:202–209.
3. Abrams P, Cardozo L, Fall M, et al. The standardisation of terminology in lower urinary tract function: report from the standardisation sub-committee of the International Continence Society. Urology 2003; 61:37–49.
4. Bright E, Cotterill N, Drake M, Abrams P. Developing and validating the International Consultation on Incontinence Questionnaire bladder diary. Eur Urol 2014; 66:294–300.
5. Martin JL, Williams KS, Abrams KR, et al. Systematic review and evaluation of methods of assessing urinary incontinence. Health Technol Assess 2006; 10:1–132.
6. Schafer W, Abrams P, Liao L, et al. Good urodynamic practices: uroflowmetry, filling cystometry, and pressure-flow studies. Neurourol Urodyn 2002; 21:261–274.
7. Hashim H, Abrams P. Is the bladder a reliable witness for predicting detrusor overactivity? J Urol 2006; 175:191–194.
8. Abrams P, Artibani W, Cardozo L, et al. Reviewing the ICS 2002 terminology report: the ongoing debate. Neurourol Urodyn 2009; 28:287.
9. Haylen BT, de Ridder D, Freeman RM, et al. An International Urogynecological Association (IUGA)/International Continence Society (ICS) joint report on the terminology for female pelvic floor dysfunction. Neurourol Urodyn 2010; 29:4–20.
10. Foon R, Toozs-Hobson P, Latthe P. Prophylactic antibiotics to reduce the risk of urinary tract infections after urodynamic studies. Cochrane Database SystRev 2012; 10:CD008224.
11. Cameron AP, Campeau L, Brucker BM, et al. Best practice policy statement on urodynamic antibiotic prophylaxis in the non-index patient. Neurourol Urodyn 2017; 36:915–926.
12. Glazener CM, Lapitan MC. Urodynamic investigations for management of urinary incontinence in adults. Cochrane Database Syst Rev 2002:CD003195.
13. Gorton E SS. Ambulatory urodynamics: do they help clinical management? BJOG 2000;107:316–319.
14. Robinson D AK, Cardozo L, Bidmead J, Toozs-Hoson P, Khullar V. Can ultrasound replace ambulatory urodynamics when investigating women with irritative urinary symptoms? BJOG 2002; 109:145–148.
15. NICE. Urinary Incontinence In Women. Clinical Guideline Cg171. London: NICE, 2013.
16. Awad SA MR. Factors that influence the incidence of detrusor instability in women. J Urol 1983; 130:114–115.
17. Serati M CE, Siesto G, Braga A, et al. Urodynamic evaluation: can it prevent the need for surgical intervention in women with apparent pure stress urinary incontinence? BJU Int 2013; 112:E344–350.
18. Radley SC, Rosario DJ, Chapple CR, Farkas AG. Conventional and ambulatory urodynamic findings in women with symptoms suggestive of bladder overactivity. J Urol 2001; 166:2253–2258.
19. Chester J, Toozs-Hobson P, Israfil-Bayli F. The role of ambulatory urodynamics in investigation of female urinary incontinence. Int Urogynecol J 2016; 27:381–386.
20. Yeung JY, Eschenbacher MA, Pauls RN. Pain and embarrassment associated with urodynamic testing in women. Int Urogynecol J 2014; 25:645–650.
21. Abrams P FR, Anderström C, Mattiasson A. Tolterodine, a new antimuscarinic agent: as effective but better tolerated than oxybutynin in patients with an overactive bladder. Br J Urol 1998; 81:801–810.
22. NICE. Urinary incontinence in neurological disease: assessment and management CG148; 2012.
23. Whiteside JL. Making sense of urodynamic studies for women with urinary incontinence and pelvic organ prolapse: a urogynecology perspective. Urol Clin North Am 2012; 39:257–263.
24. Digesu GA, Khullar V, Panayi D, et al. Should we explain lower urinary tract symptoms to patients? Neurourol Urodyn 2008; 27:368–371.
25. Wein AJ. Diagnosis and treatment of the overactive bladder. Urology 2003; 62:20–27.
26. Rachaneni S, Latthe P. Effectiveness of BTX-A and neuromodulation in treating OAB with or without detrusor overactivity: a systematic review. Int Urogynecol J 2017; 28:805–816.
27. Verghese TS ML, Daniels JP, Deeks JJ, Latthe PM. The impact of urodynamics on treatment and outcomes in women with overactive bladder: a longitudinal prospective follow up study. Int Urogynecol J 2017.
28. Suskind AM, Cox L, Clemens JQ, et al. The Value of Urodynamics in an Academic Specialty Referral Practice. Urology 2017.

29. Study N. Female Urgency, Trial of Urodynamics as Routine Evaluation (FUTURE study); a superiority randomised clinical trial to evaluate the effectiveness and cost effectiveness of invasive urodynamic investigations in management of women with refractory overactive bladder symptoms. HTA - 15/150/05, 2017.
30. Rachaneni S LP. Does preoperative urodynamics improve outcomes for women undergoing surgery for stress urinary incontinence? A systematic review and meta-analysis. BJOG 2015; 122:8–16.
31. Housley SL, Harding C, Pickard R. Urodynamic assessment of urinary incontinence. Indian J Urol 2010; 26:215–220.
32. Schierlitz L, Dwyer PL, Rosamilia A, et al. Three-year follow-up of tension-free vaginal tape compared with transobturator tape in women with stress urinary incontinence and intrinsic sphincter deficiency. Obstet Gynecol 2012; 119:321–327.
33. Brubaker L, Nygaard I, Richter HE, et al. Two-year outcomes after sacrocolpopexy with and without burch to prevent stress urinary incontinence. Obstet Gynecol 2008; 112:49–55.
34. Wei J, Nygaard I, Richter H, et al. Outcomes following vaginal prolapse repair and mid urethral sling (OPUS) trial – design and methods. Clin Trials 2009; 6:162–171.
35. van der Ploeg JM vdSA, Oude Rengerink K, van der Vaart CH, Roovers JP. Prolapse surgery with or without stress incontinence surgery for pelvic organ prolapse: a systematic review and meta-analysis of randomised trials. BJOG 2014; 121:537–547.
36. Matsuoka PK PA, Baracat EC, Haddad JM. Should prophylactic anti-incontinence procedures be performed at the time of prolapse repair? Systematic review. Int Urogynecol J 2015; 2626:187–193.
37. Srikrishna S, Robinson D, Cardozo L. Ringing the changes in evaluation of urogenital prolapse. Int Urogynecol J 2011; 22:171–175.
38. Araki I, Haneda Y, Mikami Y, Takeda M. Incontinence and detrusor dysfunction associated with pelvic organ prolapse: clinical value of preoperative urodynamic evaluation. Int Urogynecol J Pelvic Floor Dysfunct 2009; 20:1301–1306.
39. Nguyen JK, Bhatia NN. Resolution of motor urge incontinence after surgical repair of pelvic organ prolapse. JUrol 2001; 166:2263–2266.
40. Alas AN, Chinthakanan O, Espaillat L, et al. De novo stress urinary incontinence after pelvic organ prolapse surgery in women without occult incontinence. Int Urogynecol J 2017; 28:583–590.
41. Serati M, Giarenis I, Meschia M, Cardozo L. Role of urodynamics before prolapse surgery. Int Urogynecol J 2015; 26:165–168.
42. Weber AM, Walters MD. Cost-effectiveness of urodynamic testing before surgery for women with pelvic organ prolapse and stress urinary incontinence. Am J Obstet Gynecol 2000;183:1338–1346.
43. Cohn JA BE, Kaufman MR, Dmochowski RR, Reynolds WS. Underactive bladder in women: is there any evidence? Curr Opin Urol 2016; 26:309–314.
44. Sullivan JG, Swithinbank L, Abrams P. Defining achievable standards in urodynamics-a prospective study of initial resting pressures. Neurourol Urodyn 2012; 31:535–540.
45. Kraus SR, Dmochowski R, Albo ME, Xu L, Klise SR, Roehrborn CG. Urodynamic standardization in a large-scale, multicenter clinical trial examining the effects of daily tadalafil in men with lower urinary tract symptoms with or without benign prostatic obstruction. Neurourol Urodyn 2010; 29:741–747.
46. McNeil DW, Berryman ML. Components of dental fear in adults? Behav Res Ther 1989; 27:233–236.
47. Denberg TD, Melhado TV, Coombes JM, et al. Predictors of nonadherence to screening colonoscopy. J Gen Intern Med 2005; 20:989–995.
48. Yiou R, Audureau E, Loche CM, et al. Comprehensive evaluation of embarrassment and pain associated with invasive urodynamics. Neurourol Urodyn 2015; 34:156–160.
49. Rachaneni S, McCooty S, Middleton LJ, et al. Bladder ultrasonography for diagnosing detrusor overactivity: test accuracy study and economic evaluation. Health Technol Assess 2016; 20:1–150.
50. Price DD, McGrath PA, Rafii A, Buckingham B. The validation of visual analogue scales as ratio scale measures for chronic and experimental pain. Pain 1983; 17:45–56.
51. Marteau TM, Bekker H. The development of a six-item short-form of the state scale of the Spielberger State-Trait Anxiety Inventory (STAI). Br J Clin Psychol 1992; 31:301–306.
52. Latthe PM, Foon R, Toozs-Hobson P. Prophylactic antibiotics in urodynamics: a systematic review of effectiveness and safety. Neurourol Urodyn 2008; 27:167–173.
53. Gupta A, Defreitas G, Lemack GE. The reproducibility of urodynamic findings in healthy female volunteers: results of repeated studies in the same setting and after short-term follow-up. Neurourol Urodyn 2004; 23:311–316.

54. McCooty S, Nightingale P, Latthe P. The predictive value of ePAQ in the urodynamic diagnoses-A prospective cohort study. Neurourol Urodyn 2017; 37:169–176.
55. Giarenis I MP, Mastoroudes H, Robinson D, Cardozo L. Can we predict detrusor overactivity in women with lower urinary tract symptoms? The King's Detrusor Overactivity Score (KiDOS). Eur J Obstet Gynecol Reprod Biol 2016; 205:127–132.
56. Clement KD, Lapitan MC, Omar MI, Glazener CM. Urodynamic studies for management of urinary incontinence in children and adults: A short version Cochrane systematic review and meta-analysis. Neurourol Urodyn 2015; 34:407–412.

# Chapter 5

# Medical management of urinary incontinence in the premenopausal woman

*Dina El-Hamamsy, Douglas G Tincello*

## INTRODUCTION

Research studies rarely report specifically on urinary incontinence (UI) in premenopausal women. However, the prevalence of UI in this group is between 3% and 45.6% depending on the population studied, definition used in the study and whether the incontinence was bothersome [1]. These figures increase with age, pregnancy and childbirth. Other risk factors include high body mass index, smoking, caffeine and alcohol intake, and urinary tract infections (UTI).

Urinary incontinence can be divided into stress urinary incontinence (SUI) and urgency urinary incontinence (UUI). SUI is defined by the International Continence Society (ICS) as the complaint of involuntary loss of urine on effort or physical exertion, while UUI is the involuntary loss of urine associated with urgency (sudden compelling desire to void which is difficult to defer). Overactive bladder (OAB) is a syndrome including urinary urgency, usually accompanied by frequency and nocturia, with or without UUI, in absence of UTI or other obvious pathology [2].

Patients often present with symptoms of both SUI and UUI, termed mixed urinary incontinence (MUI). Other types of UI (e.g. overflow incontinence, fistula) are beyond the scope of this chapter.

Management of UI generally includes conservative, medical and surgical management. Conservative treatment for all types of incontinence includes fluid advice and management, pelvic floor muscle exercise and bladder retraining [3]. This chapter will focus on medical treatment, with reference to pregnancy and breastfeeding where data exist.

## DRUG TREATMENT

Drugs discussed here are those supported by level 1 evidence [systematic reviews, meta-analyses, or good quality randomised controlled trials (RCTs)] in women. The Oxford grades of recommendation are either A (highly recommended) or B (recommended) [4].

---

**Dina El-Hamamsy** MBBCh MSc MRCOG, Department of Health Sciences, College of Life Sciences, Univeristy of Leicester, UK

**Douglas G Tincello** BSc MBChB MD FRCOG FHEA, Department of Health Sciences, College of Life Sciences, University of Leicester, UK

## DRUGS FOR STRESS URINARY INCONTINENCE

### Duloxetine (Grade B)

This is a combined serotonin and noradrenaline re-uptake inhibitor (SNRI). It acts both centrally (on Onuf's nucleus in the sacral spinal cord) and peripherally to increases urethral sphincter activity and bladder capacity during the filling phase of micturition. It reduces incontinence episodes frequency (IEF) by up to 77% and prolongs voiding intervals (by 20 minutes versus 2 minutes for placebo), improving patients' quality of life (QoL), with up to 88% of patients feeling at least 'better' on their Global Impression of Improvement [3,5]. Duloxetine has several nonserious side effects, the commonest being nausea (25%) which subsides after 2–4 weeks. Other side effects include dyspepsia, abdominal pain, insomnia, drowsiness, headache, fatigue, and sexual dysfunction. About one in six patients discontinue treatment because of side effects [6].

Duloxetine 40 mg twice daily is licensed in the UK, Canada and Europe for treatment of moderate-to-severe SUI, and is also available in Australia, India, Bangladesh, China and South Korea. The UK National Institute for Health and Care Excellence (NICE) recommends that it is offered to women with SUI as a second line treatment option for those who prefer a pharmacological option to a surgical one [3]. The European Association of Urology (EUA) also advises dose titration on initiating treatment because of adverse events [6].

## DRUGS FOR OVERACTIVE BLADDER AND URINARY URGE INCONTINENCE

The bladder is under autonomic control mediated by the parasympathetic and the sympathetic nervous systems. The postganglionic parasympathetic neurons act via release of acetylcholine which binds to muscarinic receptors inducing bladder contraction. There are five muscarinic receptors subtypes (M1–M5). M2 is the most abundant in the detrusor muscle, although most contractile activity is mediated by M3 receptor. Muscarinic receptors are also present in the brain (M1–5), iris and ciliary muscle (M1–3), salivary glands (M1,3), heart (M2), and intestines (M3). Sympathetic control is mediated via noradrenalin neurotransmitter acting on β-adrenergic receptors. There are three β receptor subtypes, with b3 being the most abundant in human bladder, and mediates detrusor relaxation during the storage phase of micturition. Other β receptors include b1 (heart) and b2 (blood vessels) [7,8].

## ANTIMUSCARINIC DRUGS

These inhibit involuntary bladder contractions, and increase bladder capacity. They may also reduce the afferent input from the bladder during storage phase. Side effects are caused by the unwanted action on muscarinic receptors outside the bladder.

### Oxybutynin (Grade A)

Oxybutynin is considered the prototype antimuscarinic treatment for OAB, including UUI. It is a non-selective muscarinic receptor blocker that competitively inhibits the action of acetylcholine. It also has direct antispasmodic and local anaesthetic effect on the urothelium [7,8].

Oxybutynin is metabolised by the intestinal and liver cytochrome P540 enzymes into the active metabolite N-desethyloxybutynin (N-DEO) which is believed to be responsible for the majority of side effects. Caution needs to be taken in patients with hepatic or renal disease and those who have genetic heterogeneity of metabolic enzymes or taking enzyme inhibiting drugs, e.g. macrolide antibiotics, where plasma levels of the drug increase. Systemic antimuscarinic effects are a main reason for discontinuation of treatment. The commonest of these is dry mouth and the most bothersome is constipation. Other side effects include headache, somnolence, impaired cognition, and visual disturbances. Like all antimuscarinics, it is relatively contraindicated in patients with untreated closed angle glaucoma [7–9].

## Oral oxybutynin

Immediate release (IR) – Oxybutynin is effective but it may take up to 8 days to achieve maximum benefit [10]. It reduces incontinence episodes by an average of 52% with 74% mean overall improvement of OAB symptoms. However, adverse events occur in up to 88% of cases [11]. It is given as 5–20 mg/day in divided doses.

Extended/modified/sustained release oxybutynin (ER, MR, SR respectively) – use a controlled-rate drug delivery system that delivers steady amounts of the drug over 24 hours. This allows smaller amounts of the drug to be absorbed via the proximal intestine reducing the first pass hepatic metabolism. This reduces the N-DEO produced and thereby side effects. [7]. Compared to the IR, this formulation is better tolerated by patients and when objectively measured, pre-dose saliva output is maintained during its use [11]. There is a dose-dependent relationship for OAB symptoms improvement and patient satisfaction, but also for dry mouth [12]. It is given as 5–20 mg once daily.

## Non-oral oxybutynin

Non-oral preparations have been developed in an attempt to avoid the first pass hepatic metabolism and minimise systemic side effects due to N-DEO.

### Oxybutynin transdermal patch

It retains the clinical benefits of oxybutynin but with rates of dry mouth similar to placebo [13]. However, the drug delivery can be affected by skin disorders and can cause skin reactions in 11.2–35% of cases. In patients treated with oxybutynin patch, the cause of discontinuation of treatment is local rather than systemic adverse effects. The 36 mg patch releases 3.9 mg oxybutynin per day and is given twice weekly [13,14].

### Oxybutynin topical gel

It is available in two concentrations; 10% (1 g sachets) and 3% (metered-dose pump; 84 mg/day), for once daily application. It is not currently available in UK. After 12 weeks of treatment, compared to placebo, the 10% preparation reduces daily UUI (−3.0 versus −2.5, $P<0.0001$), daily micturitions (−2.7 versus −2, $P = 0.0017$), and increases voided volumes (21 versus 3.8 mL, $P = 0.0018$). The 3% gel reduces weekly UUI episodes by −20.4 (versus −18.1, $P<0.05$), daily micturitions by −2.6 (versus −1.9, $P = 0.001$) and mean voided volume (MVV) by 32.7 mL (versus 9.8 mL, $P<0.0001$) [8]. Dry mouth rate is 6.9–12.1% and skin reaction is 5.4–8.1% [7,13,14].

### Vaginal rings

Two doses of once monthly-application oxybutynin vaginal rings (4 mg/day and 6 mg/day) have been evaluated in phase 2 and 3 multicentre double blind randomised placebo controlled trials [14,15]. Compared to placebo, the mean change in weekly UUI episodes after 12 weeks treatment was −16.4 (versus −13.1, $P = 0.054$) and −16.4 ($P = 0.022$) for the 4 mg/day and 6 mg/day respectively. The dry mouth rate was 4.9–10.2% in the active drug groups, and urinary tract infections occurred in 8–11.6% of cases. Compliance was high at 99.8%. Most patients kept the ring during intercourse, although they were allowed to remove it for cleaning or if they wished to. Vaginal irritation symptoms including pain, discharge, bleeding and soreness were no different between the active drug and the placebo study groups [15,16].

## OTHER ANTIMUSCARINIC DRUGS (TABLE 5.1)

### Darifenacin (Grade A)

It is a relatively M3 selective muscarinic receptor antagonist. This in theory should reduce its systemic adverse effects, although clinically this depends on a range of factors, including pharmacokinetics and drug interactions. It is available in a long-acting once daily administration tablets (7.5–15 mg). Significant symptom improvement can be seen from second week of treatment. It improves micturition frequency, bladder capacity, frequency and severity of urgency and IEF. Improvement of nocturia is seen with the higher dose and after 12 weeks treatment. It is actively transported outside of the central nervous system (CNS) and has not been shown to produce any cardiac adverse events [7,17,18].

### Fesoterodine (Grade A)

It is a non-selective muscarinic receptor blocker that is given in doses of 4 mg or 8 mg/day. Significant improvement of OAB symptoms are seen from end of week 1 of treatment [19]. It reduces urgency and IEF, increase voided volumes and improve patients' QoL. When flexible dosing regime was used, 64% opted to increase the dose from 4–8 mg by week 8 of treatment. It is actively transported outside of the CNS and has not been shown to produce any cardiac adverse events [7,18–20].

### Solifenacin (Grade A)

It has greater affinity towards M3 than M2 receptors (more bladder specific). It is partly metabolised by the liver and partly excreted unchanged in urine. It reduces frequency, urgency, IEF, and pad use, while increasing bladder capacity and voided volumes, thereby improving patients QoL. It is given in a once daily dose of 5 mg or 10 mg. Case reports have raised concerns about prolonging cardiac QT interval in the elderly. This is not a drug class (antimuscarinic) effect, but a direct action on cardiac potassium ion channels. In extreme cases, it can lead to sudden cardiac death [18]. Although this has not been demonstrated in large post-marketing studies [7], caution needs to be taken in patients with risk factors such as hypokalaemia, bradycardia and congestive heart failure [18].

### Tolterodine (Grade A)

Although a non-selective muscarinic receptor blocker, tolterodine has greater affinity to and exerts longer lasting effects on the bladder receptors compared to salivary gland

## Table 5.1 Antimuscarinic drugs

| Drug | Oxybutynin IR | Oxybutynin ER | Darifenacin | Fesoterodine | Solifenacin | Tolterodine IR | Tolterodine ER | Trospium IR | Trospium ER | Propiverine | Imidafenacin |
|---|---|---|---|---|---|---|---|---|---|---|---|
| Efficacy (up to %) | 74% | 80% | 80% | 75% | 65% | 60% | 70% | 65% | 60% | 77% | 76% |
| Dry mouth (up to %) | 88% | 29.3% | 35.3% | 33.9 | 30% | 33% | 24.3% | 21.8% | 12.9% | 39.9% | 40.2% |
| Constipation (up to %) | 15.1% | 6.6% | 21.3% | 8.9% | 6.4% | 5.5% | 4.8% | 9.5% | 7.5% | 6.8% | 14.4% |
| CNS | Caution | | Safe | Safe | Probably safe | Caution | | Safe | | Caution | Probably safe |
| CVS | Safe | | Safe | Caution | Caution | Caution | | Safe | | Caution | Probably safe |
| FDA Pregnancy Risk Category | B | | C | C | C | C | | C | | C | Unclassified |
| Breast-feeding | Watch for poor weight gain and anticholinergic side-effects in the newborn | | | | | | | | | | |

CNS: Central nervous system. CVS: cardiovascular system. FDA drug ratings in pregnancy. B: no evidence of risk in studies, C: risk cannot be ruled out.

receptors. It is rapidly absorbed, has a half-life of 2–3 hours, and is extensively metabolised by the liver to 5HMT. Both tolterodine and 5HMT are poorly lipophilic and have limited CNS penetration ability. A small fraction of tolterodine and 5HMT is excreted in urine and may have a role acting intraluminally in the bladder. It also acts on bladder afferent pathways increasing the threshold for urgency sensation. It is given as 1–2 mg IR twice daily or 2–4 mg ER once daily doses. The extended release form has better efficacy and tolerability. Its efficacy is comparable to oxybutynin but with lower dry mouth rates. Although it does not prolong QT interval, it increases the resting heart rate by 6–10 beats/minute which can have implications in a predisposed heart or after prolonged treatment. Higher doses provide higher efficacy but at the cost of higher incidence of side effects, in keeping with all antimuscarinic drugs [7,8].

## Trospium (Grade A)

It is a non-selective muscarinic receptor blocker that does not cross the blood-brain barrier due to its large hydrophilic molecule. It is not metabolised by the hepatic P450 enzymes and is largely excreted unchanged in urine. It may act intraluminally on the bladder. It is available in short acting (20 mg twice daily) and a long acting (60 mg once daily) forms. It has proven efficacy in both idiopathic and neurogenic detrusor overactivity (DO), improving both clinical and urodynamic parameters. It reduces frequency, urgency, IEF and maximum detrusor pressure, increases bladder compliance, volume at first involuntary contraction and maximum cystometric capacity. It also improves patients' QoL. Its efficacy is comparable to oxybutynin but with better tolerability. However, it may increase the post-void residual volumes (PVR) [7,8].

## Propiverine (Grade A)

It is a smooth muscle relaxant, non-selective antimuscarinic and calcium antagonist. The latter role is yet to be proved in OAB. It is rapidly absorbed after oral administration, and has a half-life of 11–14 hours. It undergoes extensive first pass metabolism in the liver and is also a hepatic enzyme inducer. It has proven efficacy in OAB, DO (idiopathic and neurogenic) including in children. Its efficacy is comparable to oxybutynin but with less incidence and severity of dry mouth. It improves clinical and urodynamic parameters as well as patients QoL, with up to 77% subjective improvement rate. It causes voiding difficulty in about 2% of cases, however, no increase in PVR volumes has been demonstrated [7,8].

## Imidafenacin (Grade B)

This is a short-acting non-selective antimuscarinic that has greater affinity for M3 and M1 compared to M2 receptors. It is metabolised in the liver and less than 10% is excreted unchanged in the urine. It has a poorly lipophilic molecule and studies did not demonstrate cognitive concerns. It reduces urinary frequency, urgency and IEF, while increasing voided volumes and bladder capacity. It may also improve nocturia, nocturnal polyuria and nocturia-related QoL and sleep. It has not been shown to cause cardiac adverse events. Data about safety and tolerability comes from Japanese literature, so results will have to be validated in populations with other ethnicities. It is approved in Japan in a dose of 0.1 mg twice daily, which represents the best balance between efficacy and tolerability [7,8].

# SYMPATHOMIMETIC DRUGS FOR OVERACTIVE BLADDER

These are thought to act by both inhibiting detrusor contraction and reducing sensory afferents from the bladder. They increase the bladder capacity without affecting the voiding pressure or increasing PVR. Side effects are caused by the unwanted action on β-adrenergic receptors outside the bladder.

## Mirabegron (Grade B)

This is a selective b3 adrenoreceptor agonist. Compared to placebo and after 12 weeks of 50 mg treatment, it reduces daily micturitions (-1.66 versus -1.05), incontinence episodes (-1.47 versus -1.13), UUI (-1.32 versus -0.89), grade 3/4 urgency episodes (-1.57 versus -0.82), nocturia (-0.57 versus -0.38) and OAB symptom bother score (-17.0 versus -10.8), while increasing voided volumes (18.2 mL versus 7.0 mL) [21]. It is equally effective in treatment-naïve and patients who previously tried antimuscarinics. It is largely excreted unchanged in urine and stool. A smaller proportion is metabolised in the liver by two different enzymes so can be used in mild liver and moderate kidney impairment. It is generally well tolerated and discontinuation rates are low. Reported side effects include increased heart rate, increased blood pressure, and increased blood sugar, palpitations, headache, anxiety, and gastrointestinal symptoms. Hypertension and urinary tract infections are significant concerns in the elderly [1]. Mirabegron is contraindicated in severe uncontrolled hypertension (BP 180/110 mmHg), and blood pressure should be measured before starting treatment and during follow-up. NICE recommends the use of mirabegron in patients with OAB where anticholinergics are contraindicated, ineffective, or if they develop unacceptable side effects [22]. The recommended dose is 50 mg once daily (25 mg in renal or hepatic impairment).

# OTHER DRUGS

## Desmopressin (Grade A)

This is a synthetic vasopressin analogue stimulating water reabsorption in the kidney and thus reduction in urine production. It is more powerful than the natural compound and has long been used to treat nocturnal enuresis in children, and nocturia and nocturnal polyuria in adults. It is effective for treatment of urinary symptoms in multiple sclerosis (MS) and spinal cord injury patients and may have a role in daytime incontinence and other OAB symptoms. The main risk is dilutional hyponatraemia and water intoxication which can cause headache, nausea, vomiting, convulsions, or even death. This risk is greater among females, older patients and in cardiac disease. The recommended dose for idiopathic norcturnal polyuria in females in 25 µg orally one hour before bedtime (50 µg in males). For nocturia associated with MS, 10-20 µg are given intranasally at bedtime. Baseline serum sodium levels should be checked before starting treatment and repeated on third and seventh day afterwards. Patients are also advised to restrict fluid intake one hour before to 8 hours afterwards and to have their blood pressure and weight regularly checked. It should be avoided in the elderly, patients with known hyponatraemia or renal disease and those whose urine output is more than 28 mL/kg/day [7].

## Pregnancy and breastfeeding

There are few published data on the drugs mentioned above, so it is prudent to avoid the use of these drugs during pregnancy whenever possible. Available data are also limited due to small size of any studies and thus any conclusions must be interpreted with caution.

Until 2015, the US Food and Drug Administration (FDA) classified drugs in pregnancy, according to risk categories, into A (no risk), B (no evidence of risk), C (risk cannot be ruled out), D (positive evidence of risk), X (contraindicated in pregnancy).

Duloxetine is a category C drug. Small observational studies and case reports suggest it could be associated with increased risk of miscarriage but not birth defects. There are no data on preterm birth, growth restriction or child neurological development. If used near term, it may be related to poor neonatal adaptation syndrome (PNAS) which is a set of neurological symptoms due to drug withdrawal [23]. However, due to the overall paucity of safety data, duloxetine should be avoided in pregnancy. The amount of duloxetine secreted in breast milk is <1% of maternal weight-adjusted dose, which suggests it would be safe to use during breastfeeding, although there are no clinical data which confirm this [24].

Oxybutynin is a category B drug. A recent French study suggested that there was no significant increase in risk of congenital malformation following exposure in early pregnancy. However the number of study subjects was small [25]. There are no data available on the use of oxybutynin during breastfeeding. However, prolonged use might reduce milk production and the infant should be watched for poor weight gain [24].

Mirabegron is a category C drug. Data from animal studies suggest low risk in pregnancy but there are no human data. There are no reports on its use with breastfeeding [1].

Desmopresin is a category B drug. It has been safely used in cases of diabetes insipidus and Von Willebrand disease during pregnancy. The amount of desmopressin excreted in breastmilk following high dose intranasal administration is considerably less than that required to influence diuresis in infants [1].

## Combination therapy
### Combined pharmacotherapy

The concept of combined drug treatment for UI has been proposed by the International Consultation on Incontinence Research Society (ICI-RS) in 2014 [26], with a view to improving efficacy and tolerability. This is because using drugs that have different modes of action could act synergistically, and allow dose reduction of individual drugs and thereby side effects. However, combined pharmacotherapy can increase side effects, drug-drug interaction might nullify clinical effect, and the patient's overall health and cost-benefit need to be taken into account.

A combination of solifenacin and mirabegron has been tested in several studies. The SYMPHONY study showed that combined therapy improved voided volumes, micturition frequency and urgency compared to solifenacin 5 mg monotherapy. Apart from slight increase in constipation rates, no adverse events or additional safety concerns were raised [27]. The BESIDE study showed that combined therapy was superior to solifenacin 5 mg in reducing incontinence and micturition frequency and superior to solifenacin 10 mg reducing micturition frequency. Adverse events occurred in 36% of cases in the combined treatment group (33% with solifenacin 5 mg and 39% with solifenacin 10 mg). There were no increased cardiovascular or urine retention risks [28]. The MILAI study conducted in Japan demonstrated also significant reduction in OAB symptom scores by adding mirabegron to solifencin, with no safety concerns [29]. The SYNERGY study showed superiority of combined treatment over solifenacin 5 mg but not over mirabegron 50 mg monotherapies. Combined therapy resulted in slightly increased incidence of UTIs, urine retention, increased PVR, dry mouth, constipation and dyspepsia [30].

Tolterodine and pregabalin in combination have been studied in patients with idiopathic OAB. The antiepileptic pregabalin is hypothesised to act on the bladder afferent pathways more quickly and potently than its predecessor gabapentin that proved effective for NDO patients. Compared to tolterodine ER, this combination significantly improved voided volumes, micturition frequency and patients' QoL. However, pregabalin alone was also more effective than tolterodine ER or placebo improving various OAB outcomes. The commonest side effects were dry mouth and dizziness but there were no serious adverse events [26].

Desmopressin and an antimuscarinic combination has proved more successful treating nocturnal enuresis than desmopressin alone. It also proved promising in reducing number of daytime micturition and urgency episodes in OAB patients, and improving their QoL [21].

## Treatment pathways for OAB

Failing conservative therapy, and before embarking on invasive treatment, patients should be offered pharmacological treatment. Principles of pharmacotherapy include offering the lowest effective dose, titrating dose according to response/side effects profile, allowing enough time (usually 4 weeks) for the therapeutic effect to take place followed by clinical review to evaluate benefit and need for drug change. Caution needs to be taken when assessing the women's overall condition (e.g. voiding difficulty) and concomitant medication (drug interactions and anticholinergic burden). Most antimuscarinics have comparable side effects which can usually be managed conservatively (e.g. saliva replacement for dry mouth and laxatives for constipation). Long acting and non-oral formulations are generally better tolerated by patients.

The NICE recommends starting treatment by IR oxybutynin/ tolterodine or darifenacin, failing which another antimuscarinic with the lowest acquisition cost should be offered. Transdermal oxybutynin is offered in cases of good efficacy but poor tolerability of oral oxybutynin. Mirabegron is offered if antimuscarinics are not effective, not tolerated or contra-indicated [4]. According to EAU and American Urological Association, however, mirabegron may also be offered to patients failing conservative management without trying antimuscarincs [7,31].

Failure of therapy with two or more antimuscarinic drugs and mirabegron would be an indication to consider invasive second line therapy including botulinum toxin injection to the bladder wall, via cystoscopy or sacral nerve modulation via implantable electrodes.

## ANTICHOLINERGIC BURDEN

Patients' who are prescribed anti muscarinic treatment for OAB may need to take other medications that have anticholinergic activity. These include drugs given primarily for their anticholinergic action (e.g. antiemetics and antispasmodics), or those with anticholinergic side effects (e.g. some antihistamines and antidepressants).

The cumulative effect of taking one or more drugs with anticholinergic properties, the "anticholinergic burden", is related to the number of drugs taken and the duration they have been used for. Attempts have been made to grade the clinical and biochemical anticholinergic effect of various medications to try and reduce the anticholinergic burden of prescribing. According to clinical scales, the anticholinergic activity of a drug can be low (e.g. ampicillin, citalopram and metformin), moderate (e.g. baclofen, ocarbazepine and methadone) or high (e.g. amitriptyline, chlorpheniramine and chlorpromazine) [32].

There is an abundance of muscarinic receptors in the brain, with M1 being particularly important in higher cognitive functions such as learning and memory. There is also growing evidence that high ACB can affect cognitive functions, with concerns that these changes might not be reversible on stopping anticholinergic medications. There is also objective evidence of reduced hippocampus glucose metabolism and cortical brain atrophy in anticholinergic users.

A recent study showed that 23% of patients on anticholinergic drugs developed dementia when followed for a mean of 7.3 years (80% Alzheimer disease), with a 10-year cumulative dose-response relationship [33]. Risk factors for overall cognitive impairment include age, sex, number of drugs and ACB score. When individual brain functions were studied, episodic memory (memory of facts and emotions of particular events) was particularly affected and this was independent of age, sex, education, depression and cardiovascular risk or disease.

Although evidence comes from the elderly population on polypharmacy, as patients present at a younger age, the potential of being on anticholinergic drugs for longer exists, increasing the anticholinergic burden and risk. The new emergence of non-anticholinergic treatments of OAB should reduce such risk. However, this potential risk of long term cognitive dysfunction in patients taking anticholinergic drugs for long periods should be discussed with patients before initiating prescription. The precise risk from antimuscarinic drugs alone in young adults has not yet been fully quantified.

### Key points for clinical practice

- Duloxetine should be offered as a second line treatment for patients with SUI who prefer a pharmacological option after counselling about side effects.
- Antimuscarinic drugs are all equally effective in management of OAB symptoms, but side effects limit their tolerability.
- Long acting and non-oral preparations improve anticholinergic tolerability.
- Mirabegron avoids antimuscarinic side effects and is a useful alternative drug. Caution with hypertension.
- Desmopressin is used for treatment of nocturia, nocturnal polyuria and enuresis. Caution with hyponatraemia.
- Combination therapy may improve clinical outcomes without posing significant safety risks.
- High anticholinergic burden increases risk of cognitive impairment/ dementia which may not be reversible. The precise risk is not yet quantified.

# REFERENCES

1. Minassian VA, Yan X, Lichtenfeld MJ, Sun H, Stewart WF. The iceberg of health care utilization in women with urinary incontinence. Int Urogynecol J 2012; 23:1087–93.
2. Haylen BT, Ridder D, Freeman RM, et al. IUGA/ICS Joint Report On The Terminology For Female Pelvic Floor Dysfunction. Neurourol Urodyn 2010; 29:4–20.

3. National Institute for Health and Care Excellence. Urinary incontinence in women: management. Clinical guideline (CG171) 2015.
4. Andersson KE, et al. Pharmacological treatment of urinary incontinence. In: Abrams P, et al., editors. Incontinence, 5th international consultation on incontinence, ICUD-EAU; 2013:623–728.
5. Li J, Yang L, Pu C, et al. The role of duloxetine in stress urinary incontinence: a systematic review and meta-analysis. Int Urol Nephrol 2013; 45:679–686.
6. European Association of Urology. Urinary incontinence guideline, 2016.
7. Smith AL, Wein AJ. Drug treatment of lower urinary tract dysfunction in women. In: CardozoL, Staskin D, editors. Textbook of female urology and urogynaecology. Fourth edition. Boca Raton: CRC Press; 2017:515–550.
8. Andersson K-E, Wein AJ. Pharmacologic management of lower urinary tract storage and emptying failure. In: Wein AJ (Ed) Campbell-Walsh Urology, eleventh edition 2016; 1836–1874.
9. Jirschele K, Sand PK. Oxybutynin: past, present, and future. Int Urogynecol J 2013; 24:595–604.
10. Herschorn S, Pomerville P, Stothers L, et al. Tolerability of Solifenacin and oxybutynin immediate release in older (>65 years) and younger (<65 years).
11. Chancellor MB, Appell RA, Sathyan G, Gupta SK. A comparison of the effects on saliva output of oxybutynin chloride and tolterodine tartrate. Clin Ther 2001; 23:753.
12. Corcos J, Casey R, Patrick A, et al. A double-blind randomized dose- response study comparing daily doses of 5, 10 and 15 mg controlled- release oxybutynin: balancing efficacy with severity of dry mouth. BJU Int 2006; 97:520–527.
13. Cartwright R, Srikrishna S, Cardozo L, Robinson D. Patient-selected goals in overactive bladder: a placebo controlled randomized double-blind trial of transdermal oxybutynin for the treatment of urgency and urge incontinence. BJU Int 2011; 107:70–76.
14. Cohn JA, Brown ET, Reynolds WS, et al. An update on the use of transdermal oxybutynin in the management of overactive bladder disorder. Therapeutic Advances in Urology 2016; 8:83–90.
15. Gittelman M, Weiss H, Seidman L. A phase 2, randomized, double-blind, efficacy and safety study of oxybutynin vaginal ring for alleviation of overactive bladder symptoms in women. J Urol 2014; 191:1014–1021.
16. Swierzewski M, Seidman L, Dasen S, Weiss H. Phase 3 efficacy and safety of once-monthly oxybutynin vaginal ring delivering 4mg/day or 6mg/day vs placebo ring in women with urge incontinence, frequency, and urgency symptoms of overactive bladder. J Urol 2013; 189:E232.
17. Khullar V, Foote J, Seifu Y, Egermark M. Time-to-effect with darifenacin in overactive bladder: a pooled analysis 2011; 22:1573–1580.
18. Kowey PR. Cardiovascular risks of anticholinergic therapy: considerations for office-based management. OBG Management 2007; 19:S7–10.
19. Wagg A, Khullar V, Marschall-Kehrel D, et al. Flexible-dose fesoterodine in elderly adults with overactive bladder: results of the randomised double-blind placebo-controlled study of fesoterodine in an aging population trial. JAGS 2013; 61:185–193.
20. Goldman HB, Morrow JD, Gong J, Tseng LJ, Schneider T. Early onset of fesoterodine efficacy in subjects with overactive bladder. BJUI 2010; 107:598–602.
21. Nitti VW, Auerbach S, Martin N, Calhoun A, Lee M, Herschorn S. Results of a randomised phase III trial of Mirabegron in patients with overactive bladder. Journal of Urology 2013;189:1388–1395.
22. National Institute for Health and Care Ecellence. Mirabegron for treating symptoms of overactive bladder. Technology appraisal guidance (TA290), 2013.
23. Andrade C. The safety of duloxetine during pregnancy and lactation. J Clin Psychiatry 2014; 75:e1423.
24. Toxicology data network, US National Library of Medicine (cited 25th April 2017). Available from https://toxnet.nlm.nih.gov/newtoxnet/lactmed.htm
25. Beghin D, Vauzelle-Gardier C, Elefant E. Pregnancy outcome after in utero exposure to oxybutynin. Reproductive Toxicology 2016; 60:177–178.
26. Visco AG, Fraser MO, Newgreen D, et al. What is the role of combination drug therapy in the treatment of overactive bladder? ICI-RS 2014. Neurourol Urodynam 2016; 35: 288–292.
27. Abrams P, Kelleher C, Staskin D, et al. Combination treatment with mirabegron and solifenacin in patients with overactive bladder (OAB) - efficacy and safety results from a randomised phase II study (SYMPHONY). Neurourology and Urodynamics 2013; 32:930–931.
28. Drake MJ, Chapple C, Esen AA, et al. Efficacy and Safety of mirabegron add-on therapy to solifenacin in incontinent overactive bladder patients with an inadequate response to initial 4-week solifenacin monotherapy: a randomised double-blind multi centre phase 3B study (BESIDE). European Urology 2016; 70:136–145.

29. Yamaguchi O, Kakizaki H, Homma Y, et al. Safety and efficacy of mirabegron as 'add-on' therapy in patients with overactive bladder treated with solifenacin: a post-marketing open-label study in Japan (MILAI study). BJU Int 2015; 116:612–622.
30. Herschorn S, Chapple C, Abrams P, et al. Efficacy and safety of combinations of mirabegron and solifenacin compared with monotherapy and placebo in patients with overactive bladder (SYNERGY study). BJU Int. 2017; accepted for publication.
31. American Urological Association. Diagnosis and Treatment of Non-Neurogenic Overactive Bladder (OAB) in Adults: AUA/SUFU Guideline - (2012, 2014).
32. Salahudeen MS, Duffull SB, Nishtala PS. Anticholinergic burden quantified by anticholinergic risk scales and adverse outcomes in older people: a systematic review. BMC Geriatrics 2015:15–31.
33. Gray SL, Anderson ML, Dublin S, et al. Cumulative use of strong anticholinergics and incident dementia, a prospective study. JAMA Intern Med 2015; 175:401–407.

# Chapter 6

# Caesarean scar ectopic pregnancy

*Venetia Goodhart, Davor Jurkovic*

## INTRODUCTION

The rate of caesarean sections as a mode of delivery has significantly increased in developed countries over recent decades. The rate ranges between 6.2% and 36% with an average of 21.1% [1]. This change has naturally been accompanied by an increase in the rates of complications associated with this form of surgical intervention. Adverse effects associated with a history of previous caesarean section include scar dehiscence, uterine rupture, abnormal placentation (placenta previa and accreta), post-operative pelvic adhesions and the development of a deficient caesarean section scar [2,3]. Risk factors for development of deficient caesarean section scars are thought to be uterine retroflexion, multiple caesarean sections and single layer closure of the myometrium, with 19.4% of women with previous caesarean sections affected [2,3]. These deficient caesarean section scars are thought to facilitate the development of caesarean section scar pregnancies.

The term caesarean section scar pregnancy refers to a type of ectopic pregnancy, defined by the implantation of the gestational sac completely or partially outside the uterine cavity into the previous lower uterine segment caesarean section scar [3]. These pregnancies have been shown to be associated with severe haemorrhage due to abnormally adherent placentas and loss of functional myometrium at the implantation site The aim of this chapter is to further understand the importance of identifying these pregnancies, their associated risk factors, diagnostic criteria using ultrasound scanning, and management.

## INCIDENCE, RISK FACTORS AND PRESENTATION

Although, caesarean section scar (CS) ectopic pregnancies are relatively rare, they carry significant risks of complications and should be identified and managed appropriately, and in a timely manner. caesarean scar ectopic pregnancies occur in approximately 1 in 1,800 pregnancies [4,5]. However, in women with a history of two or more caesarean sections, the risk can be as high as 1 in 50 pregnancies. The increased incidence of CS pregnancies can be attributed to the increased rates of CS but can also be explained by the liberal use of transvaginal scan in the first trimester and the development of clear ultrasound diagnostic criteria.

---

**Venetia Goodhart** BSc MBBS, Department of Obstetrics and Gynaecology, University College London Hospital, London, UK

**Davor Jurkovic** MD PhD FRCOG, Institute for Women's Health, Faculty of Population Health Sciences, University College London (UCL), London

## Risk factors

The major contributing factor for the development of a CS ectopic pregnancy is poor healing of the previous caesarean section scar, described using a range of terms. These include caesarean scar defect, deficient caesarean scar, pouch, isthmocele, diverticulum and niche [2]. Risk factors for suboptimal healing were shown to include single layer closure of the myometrium, a history of multiple caesarean sections and retroflexion of the uterus [2,6]. In the UK 96% of the UK's obstetricians use a double layer closure for lower uterine segment caesarean sections, but there are considerable variations in the closure technique worldwide [7]. The pathophysiology of multiple Cesarean sections contributing to scar defects has been explained by the observation that recurrent trauma to the same area can impair normal healing [8]. Ofili-Yebovi et al. [3] explored the theory that as the CS scar is at the level of the internal os and that this is the flexion point of the uterus, retroflexion therefore causes a degree of tension at this point.

A study examining deficient Cesarean section scars reported that 32 of the 324 women examined (9.9%, 95% CI 7.1 to 13.4) had severe lower uterine segment scar defects, with $\geq$ 50% myometrial involvement [3]. Vikhareva Osser et al. [6] concluded that there is no direct association between larger scar defects seen at transvaginal ultrasound and increased risks of complications in future pregnancies such as CS ectopic pregnancies, abnormal placentation, uterine rupture and scar dehiscence.

As with any type of ectopic pregnancy, a caesarean scar ectopic pregnancy is located outside the uterine cavity – defined as the virtual space lined with endometrium between the internal cervical os and the ostia of the Fallopian tubes. The pregnancy is implanted in the deficient lower uterine segment caesarean section scar and the gestational sac is either partially or completely within the myometrial mantle. There must be evidence of functional peri-trophoblastic flow on colour Doppler examination [9].

A poorly healed lower segment uterine caesarean scar lacks decidua. This absence of normal architecture at the level of the scar allows the trophoblast to invade into the myometrium between the fibres of the uterine muscle, potentially extending into the bladder or uterine serosa [10]. As a result of implantation occurring where the vasculature is not suited to support the developing pregnancy, the placenta becomes abnormally adherent as it extends into the myometrium in search of nutrition [9]. Low oxygen tension in a local area (e.g. a CS scar site) has been identified as an important factor in the invasion of the cytotrophoblast and its proliferation in order to regulate placentation [11].

## Presentation

Whilst caesarean scar ectopics can be asymptomatic and be diagnosed incidentally, many will present with bleeding or pain in the first trimester. Fabres et al. [12] reported that 76% of women diagnosed with a niche at the site of the previous CS scar experienced abnormal uterine bleeding such as postmenstrual spotting (**Figure 6.1**).

### Diagnostic importance and criteria

Severe bleeding in early pregnancy can be associated with a range of diagnoses and is not exclusive to CS ectopic pregnancies. Other causes for excessive bleeding include prolonged retained products of conception (RPOC), late first trimester miscarriage as well as cervical ectopic pregnancy. Approximately 50% of CS ectopics will miscarry in the first and second trimesters and those that do progress tend to develop abnormally adherent placentas resulting in placenta previa or accreta [3,4,13]. As a result of abnormal placentation,

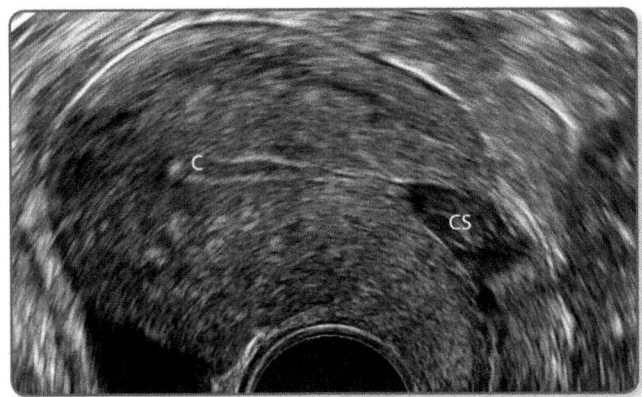

**Figure 6.1** Cesarean scar defect. A retroflexed uterus with an empty uterine cavity (C) and a deficient Cesarean section scar (CS). The defect has a thin layer of myometrium anteriorly. Blood collecting in this defect during menstruation can present as postmenstrual spotting.

placental separation is affected. Combined with the absence of functional myometrium, resulting in poor uterine contraction, the difficulty in placental separation can result in maternal haemorrhage.

Timor-Tritsch et al. [10] compared the placental histology between early placenta accreta (visible in the second trimester) and that of CS pregnancies. They established that the histological features were indistinguishable and hypothesized that they are early demonstrations of morbidly adherent placenta; that CS pregnancies can be considered as a precursor of morbidly adherent placenta. Furthermore, Wu et al. [14] found that the risk of faulty placentation increases with the increase in the number of caesarean sections.

Abnormal placental adherence has been shown by Bij de Vaate et al. [2] to be a major contributing factor for obstetric hysterectomy, accounting for 41–64% of cases. The majority of these patients had a history of previous caesarean section.

Clear diagnostic criteria using transvaginal ultrasound have been established in order to help clinicians identify this potential complication in early pregnancy. Transvaginal ultrasonography is well suited for identifying the diagnostic features of CS ectopic pregnancies, which are as follows:

- The pregnancy is partially or completely outside the uterine cavity on transvaginal ultrasound examination. The cavity should be carefully examined in transverse and longitudinal sections to confirm the absence of an intracavitary pregnancy and the endometrial thickness should be measured and recorded. In some women, the gestational sac is partially extrauterine invading the broad ligament or entering the vesico-uterine pouch
- The CS ectopic pregnancy implants into the anterior wall of the uterus at the level of the previous lower uterine caesarean section scar. This is at the level of, or below the level of the internal cervical os, breeching the endometrial myometrial junction. Involvement of the myometrium is further evidenced in cases of herniation of the pregnancy, usually anteriorly towards the bladder or the broad ligament (**Figure 6.2**) [9]
- Demonstration of functional peri-trophoblastic or placental circulation. This occurs anteriorly to the gestational sac or solid mass of trophoblast [15] on colour Doppler examination, confirming implantation within the deficient scar [9] (**Figure 6.3**)
- The 'sliding organ sign' is negative. When gentle pressure is applied using the transvaginal ultrasound probe, the gestational sac is fixed in position and cannot be displaced from its location at the level of the previous caesarean section scar

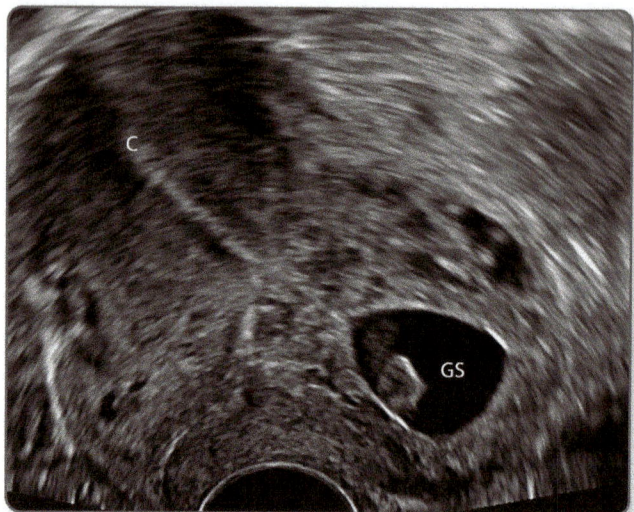

**Figure 6.2** Anterior herniation of a Cesarean scar pregnancy. The uterine cavity (C) is empty and the gestational sac (GS) and overlying myometrium are herniating towards the bladder.

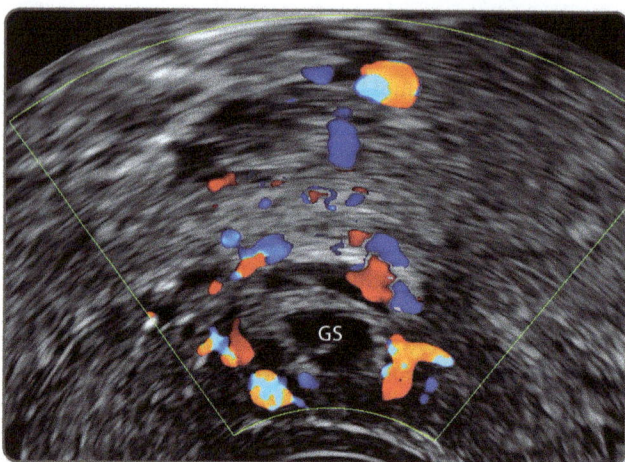

**Figure 6.3** Vascular supply of a Cesarean scar pregnancy. Functional peri-trophoblastic circulation is demonstrated using colour Doppler examination and is displayed anterior to the gestational sac (GS) and within the Cesarean section scar.

## Assessing vascularity

Assessment of the vascularity, while not associated with risk of haemorrhage in a normal myometrium, can provide an indication of the risk of severe bleeding in CS ectopic pregnancies. The insufficient myometrium, in these cases of deficient lower uterine segment Cesarean section scars, does not hold the ability to contract as expected, contributing to blood loss. Vascularity is proportional to haemorrhage risk in CS ectopic pregnancies (**Table 6.1**) [16]. These pregnancies are associated with an increased risk of spontaneous haemorrhage as well as haemorrhage at surgical evacuation. This factor plays an important role in decisions around best management. Advancing gestational age is also associated with increased complications and blood loss [17,18]. Using 3D ultrasound to aid diagnosis of CS ectopic pregnancies.

The primary use of 3D ultrasound in gynaecology is in the identification and demonstration of congenital and acquired uterine anomalies. In addition, 3D imaging has

Table 6.1 Association between vascularity and associated blood loss of CS pregnancies with permission from Jurkovic et al. [16]

| Vascularisation | Estimated blood loss (IQR) |
|---|---|
| No vascularity (1) | 50 mL (50 mL – 100 mL) |
| Minimal (2) | 100 mL (50 mL – 300 mL) |
| Moderate (3) | 200 mL (100 mL – 375 mL) |
| High (4) | 300 mL (175 mL – 1,350 mL) |
| N = 190 | |

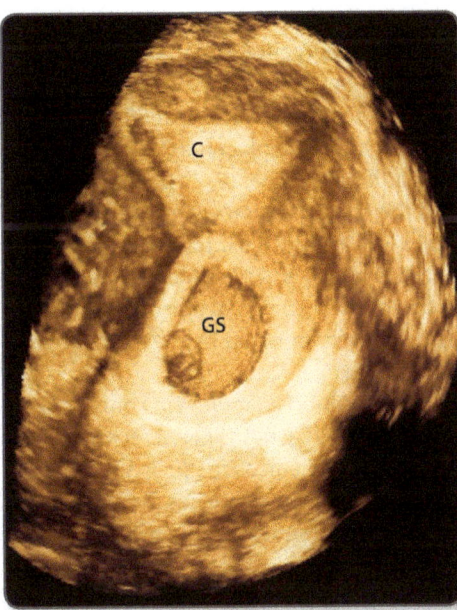

**Figure 6.4** Coronal view in 3D of a Cesarean scar pregnancy. The gestation sac (GS) sits below the uterine cavity (C) in the coronal view and demonstrates breeching of the endometrial myometrial junction.

the ability to clearly exhibit the endometrial myometrial junction, supplementing standard B-mode imaging [19]. This function allows clinicians to further examine the location of the pregnancy in relation to the uterine cavity and whether the endometrial myometrial junction has been breeched. CS ectopic pregnancies do breech this junction and involve the myometrium (**Figure 6.4**), which results in a partial or absent decidual reaction. As well as playing a role in diagnosis, 3D imaging allows clinicians to ascertain the degree of myometrial involvement, and whether surgical evacuation is likely to be feasible or not. By confirming the site of the pregnancy with the assistance of 3D ultrasound, clinicians can establish the best route for surgical management – transabdominal or transvaginal.

## Differential diagnoses

Differential diagnoses for a caesarean section scar ectopic pregnancy on ultrasound include cervical ectopic pregnancies as well as the cervical stage of an ongoing miscarriage [9]. Colour Doppler can be employed to differentiate between these diagnoses. A scar ectopic will typically demonstrate increased vascularity on colour Doppler examination, in its anterior aspect and within the previous caesarean section scar. In contrast, the vascularity of a cervical ectopic pregnancy will be usually posteriorly within the cervical canal. During the cervical phase of an ongoing miscarriage, the gestational sac may overly the previous CS scar, which raises the suspicion of a CS ectopic pregnancy. Colour Doppler examination enables the clinician to identify the implantation site. Although the gestational sac may lie adjacent to the CS scar, the placental implantation site will be superior to the sac and within the uterine cavity or posterior to the gestational sac (**Figure 6.5**). In these cases, the pregnancy may overlie the previous caesarean scar but implantation posterior to the gestational sac excludes the diagnosis of a CS ectopic pregnancy.

**Reproductive outcomes and recurrence**
Reproductive outcomes of women with a history of previous CS ectopic pregnancy were examined in 2007. Out of the 40 patients managed, 2 had emergency hysterectomies (5%, 95% CI: 0–12). Both had had expectant management and one had a spontaneous miscarriage at 17 weeks, whilst the other had an elective caesarean section at 38 weeks. Both had severe haemorrhage secondary to abnormally adherent placentas [20]. When looking at possible predictive indicators of morbidly adherent placenta, Zosmer et al. [15] found that if the majority of the placental tissue and the cord insertion were in the scar defect on ultrasound in the first trimester and if there was evidence of herniation, women were more likely to experience massive obstetric haemorrhage and possible hysterectomy. Placental lakes detected on ultrasound in the first trimester are a sign of placental dysfunction, seen more commonly in CS pregnancies, which therefore help to confirm the diagnosis.

Following successful treatment of CS 95% (95% CI: 86–100) of women who conceived again had intrauterine pregnancies and one woman (5%, 95% CI: 0–14) had a recurrence of CS ectopic pregnancy. Ben Nagi et al. [20] felt that this low recurrence rate is suggestive that recurrence is more likely due to chance. Similar low recurrence rate has also been reported when looking at the efficacy and safety of ultrasound-guided suction curettage of CS ectopic pregnancies [16].

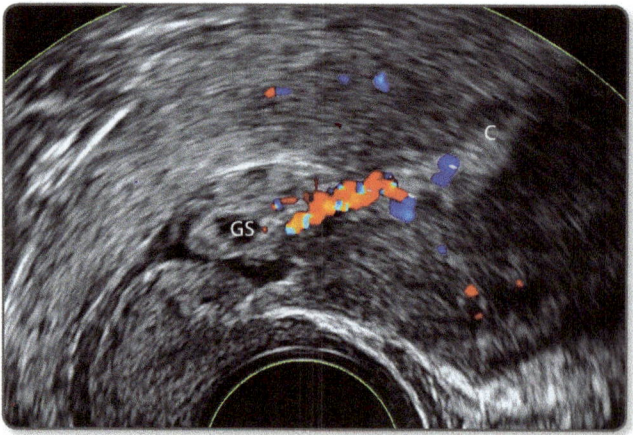

**Figure 6.5** Ongoing miscarriage. The gestational sac (GS) overlies the Cesarean section scar. However, colour Doppler examination demonstrates implantation in the uterine cavity (C).

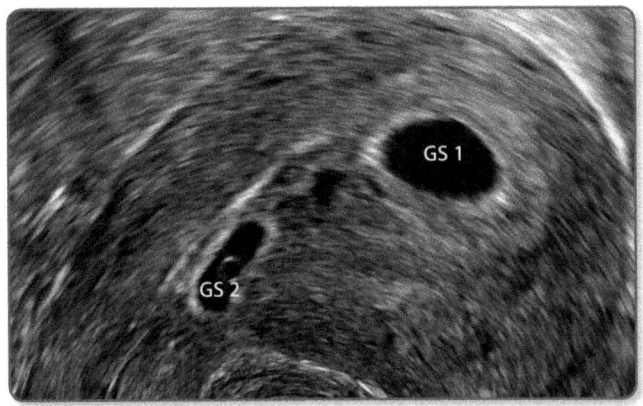

**Figure 6.6** Heterotopic CS pregnancy. A gestational sac is seen within the uterine cavity as well as a gestational sac (GS 1) implanted within the Cesarean section scar (GS 2).

## Heterotopic caesarean scar pregnancies

Rates of heterotopic pregnancies (**Figure 6.6**) have risen with the development of assisted reproduction and are now thought to be approximately 1% [21,22]. A review by OuYang et al. [23] identified 14 cases of heterotopic CS ectopic pregnancies. Eight of the 14 cases were conceived through IVF and embryo transfer, and the remainder conceived spontaneously. Thirteen chose to preserve the intrauterine pregnancy and 12 underwent intervention, whilst one had expectant management. One had a termination for fetal abnormalities and of the 12 remaining; all had live births via caesarean sections. Four had massive obstetric haemorrhage and one required a hysterectomy [23]. Those that opt for selective termination tend to have good outcomes.

**Management** Specific understanding of the exact location of the CS ectopic pregnancy, its size and vascularity can aid clinicians in establishing tailored management plans for patients. The diagnosis and potential complications should be clearly explained to patients to enable them to make informed decisions about management. Decisions regarding timing and type of management are also affected by the gestational age of the pregnancy, its viability, the patients' symptoms and the degree of myometrial deficiency [24]. Management options include expectant management, medical management and surgical management.

Expectant management of live scar pregnancies carries significant risks and is associated with high maternal morbidity following the development of morbidly adherent placentas. 70% will incur massive obstetric haemorrhage and 50% require emergency hysterectomy [15]. Medical management with the administration of methotrexate succeeds in approximately 50% of cases [9]. Surgical management in the form of transvaginal surgical evacuation can be performed with or without the insertion of a Shirodkar cervical suture or Foley catheter as an aid to prevent maternal haemorrhage [16]. This form of management carries fewer risks – 5% risk of blood transfusion and <1% risk of hysterectomy if additional measures fail and is successful in 92–96% of cases [9,15].

The median time to resolution is 2 months in cases that undergo successful medical management. Transvaginal ultrasound can be used following expectant, medical or surgical management to assess for resolution of the scar pregnancy. Abnormal vaginal bleeding following management may indicate retained products of conception and should be assessed with ultrasound.

## CONCLUSION

Clear diagnostic criteria using ultrasound have been established as a safe and effective method of identifying Cesarean scar pregnancies in the first trimester. Although some have suggested that routine screening for Cesarean scar pregnancies should be carried out, such a policy is of unproven value with a significant risk of both false positive and false negative findings [25]. However, an early scan at 6-7 weeks' gestation could be considered in women with previous history of scar pregnancies and those with a past history of multiple Cesarean sections [3].

> **Key points for clinical practice**
> - Women with a history of previous caesarean section, who present with suspected complications in early pregnancy (abdominal pain or vaginal bleeding), should be assessed with transvaginal ultrasound.
> - Early diagnosis enables timely and appropriate management.
> - Diagnosis is based on:
>   - An empty uterine cavity
>   - Evidence of a breech of the endometrial-myometrial junction at, or below the level of the internal cervical os
>   - Functional peri-trophoblastic flow anterior to the gestational sac
>   - A negative 'sliding organ sign'
> - Differential diagnoses are cervical ectopic pregnancy and the cervical phase of miscarriage.
> - CS ectopic pregnancies are associated with severe haemorrhage secondary to abnormal placentation, either spontaneously but more commonly at surgical evacuation.
> - Management options include expectant, medical and surgical management.
> - Assessment of the vascularity of the pregnancy and 3D assessment helps to establish the bleeding risk and feasibility of surgical evacuation.
> - If patients wish to continue with the pregnancy, in cases of viable CS ectopic pregnancies, the risks must be fully explained and cases should be referred to fetal medicine colleagues for continued assessment for placenta previa or accreta.
> - Transvaginal ultrasound should be used to assess for RPOC in women with abnormal bleeding following management of CS ectopic pregnancies.
> - In the absence of local expertise, cases should be discussed with, or referred to a specialist centre for diagnosis and management.

## REFERENCES

1. Betrán AP, Merialdi M, Lauer JA, et al. Rates of caesarean section: analysis of global, regional and national estimates. Paediatr Perinat Epidemiol 2007; 21:98–113.
2. Bij de Vaate AJM, Ven der Voet LF, Naji O, et al. Prevalence, potential risk factors for development and symptoms related to the presence of uterine niches following Cesarean section: systematic review. Ultrasound Obstet Gynecol 2014; 43:372–382.
3. Ofili-Yebovi D, Ben-Nagi J, Sawyer E et al. Deficient lower-segment Cesarean section scars: prevalence and risk factors. Ultrasound Obstet Gynecol 2008; 31:72–77.

4. Jurkovic D, Hillaby K, Woelfer B, et al. First trimester diagnosis and management of pregnancies implanted into the lower uterine segment caesarean section scar. Ultrasound Obstet Gynaecol 2003; 21:220–227
5. Seow K, Huang L, Lin Y, et al. caesarean scar pregnancy: issues in management. Ultrasound Obstet Gynaecology 2004; 23:247–253
6. Vikhareva Osser O, Jokubkiene L, Valentin L. High prevalence of defects in Cesarean section scars at transvaginal ultrasound examination. Ultrasound Ostet Gynecol 2009; 34:90–97
7. Tulley L, Gates S, Brocklehurst P, et al. Surgical techniques used during caesarean section operations: results of a national survey of practice in the UK, Eur J Obstet Gynecol Reprod Biol, 2002, vol. 102 (pg. 120–126).
8. Wound healing, chronic wounds http://www.emedicine.com/plastic/topic477.htm
9. Harb HM, Knight M, Bottomley C, et al. caesarean scar pregnancy in the UK: a national cohort study. BJOG. 2018; 125:1663–1670.
10. Timor-Tritsch IE, Monteagudo G, Cali G, et al. Cesarean scar pregnancy and early placenta accrete share common histology. Ultrasound Obstet Gynecol 2014; 43:383–395
11. Genbacev O, Zhou Y, Ludlow JW, et al. Regulation of human placental development be oxygen tension. Science 1997; 277:1669–1672.
12. Fabres C, Aviles G, De La Jara C, et al. The cesarean delivery scar pouch: clinical implications and diagnostic correlation between transvaginal sonography and hysteroscopy. J Ultrasound Med 2003; 22:695–700.
13. Ben Nagi J, Ofili-Yebovi D, Marsh M, Jurkovic D. First trimester Cesarean scar pregnancy evolving into placenta previa/accreta at term. J Ultrasound Med 2005; 24:1569–73.
14. Wu S, Kocherginsky M, Hibbard JU. Abnormal placentation: twenty-year analysis. Am J Obstet Gynecol 2005; 192: 1458–1461.
15. Zosmer N, Fuller J, Shaikh H, et al. Natural history of early first-trimester pregnancies implanted in Cesarean scars. Ultrasound Obstet Gynecol. 2015 Sep;46(3):367-75. doi: 10.1002/uog.14775. Epub 2015 Aug 6.
16. Jurkovic D, Knez J, Appiah A, et al. Surgical treatment of Cesarean scar ectopic pregnancy: Efficacy and safety of ultrasound-guided suction curettage. Ultrasound Obstet Gynecol 2016 Apr;47(4):511–7.
17. Jurkovic D, Ben Nagi J, Ofili-Yebovi D, et al. Efficacy of Shirodkar cervical suture in securing hemostasis following surgical evacuation of Cesarean scar ectopic pregnancy. Ultrasound Obstet Gynecol 2007; 30:95–100.
18. Van den Bosch T, Van Schoubroeck D, Timmerman D. Maximum Peak Systolic Velocity and Management of Highly Vascularized Retained Products of Conception. J Ultrasound Med. 2015 Sep;34(9):1577–82.
19. Naftalin J, Hoo W, Nunes N, et al. Inter- and intraobserver variability in three-dimensional ultrasound assessment of the endometrial-myometrial junction and factors affecting its visualization. Ultrasound Obstet Gynecol 2012;39(5):587-91. Doi:10.1002/uog.10133.
20. Ben Nagi J, Helmy S, Ofili-Yebovi D, et al. Reproductive outcomes of women with a previous history of caesarean scar ectopic pregnancies. Hum Reprod 2007; 22(7): 2012–2015.
21. Salomon LJ, Fernandez H, Chauveaud A, et al. Successful management of a heterotopic caesarean scar pregnancy: potassium chloride injection with preservation of the intrauterine gestation— case report. Hum Reprod 2003; 18:189–191.
22. Wang CN, Chen CK, Wang HS, et al. Successful management of heterotopic caesarean scar pregnancy combined with intrauterine pregnancy after in vitro fertilization–embryo transfer. Fertil Steril 2007; 88:706.e13–706.e16.
23. OuYang Z, Yin Q, Xu Y, et al. Heterotopic Cesarean scar pregnancy: Diagnosis, Treatment and Prognosis. J Ultrasound Med 2014; 33:1533–1537.
24. Jurkovic D, Hillaby K, Woelfer B, et al. First trimester diagnosis and management of pregnancies implanted into the lower uterine segment Cesarean section scar. Ultrasound Obstet Gynecol 2003; 21:220–27.
25. Timor-Tritsch IE, D'Antonio F, Cali G, Palacios-Jaraquemada J, Meyer J, Monteagudo A. Early first trimester transvaginal ultrasound is indicated in pregnancies after a previous cesarean delivery: should it be mandated? Ultrasound Obstet Gynecol. 2019 Jan 24. doi: 10.1002/uog.20225. [Epub ahead of print]

# Chapter 7

# Ambulatory interventions in the management of acute gynaecology and early pregnancy complications

*Kim Lawson, Cecilia Bottomley*

## INTRODUCTION

Ambulatory care is the streamlined approach to diagnosis and management of patients who traditionally would have been admitted to a hospital bed. This has broad advantages both to hospital care providers where costs are minimised by keeping patients at home, but also to patients who maintain social functioning by avoiding hospital admission.

There is a rapid expansion in emergency ambulatory care for all specialties, with networks and support programmes developed to provide the training, resources and support to facilitate healthcare teams in maximising the impact of this pathway [1].

Ambulatory interventions in common use in acute gynaecology and early pregnancy care are summarised in **Table 7.1**. In some cases care might involve a 'one-stop' visit

| \multicolumn{2}{c}{Table 7.1 Ambulatory interventions in common use in acute gynaecology and early pregnancy settings} | |
|---|---|
| Acute gynaecology | Outpatient management of hyperemesis |
| | Word catheter for Bartholin's cyst/abscess |
| | Outpatient drainage of pelvic abscess or cyst |
| | Drainage of haematometra/pyometra |
| | Hysteroscopic interventions (e.g. retrieval of lost IUCD) |
| | Ambulatory intravenous antibiotics for pelvic infection |
| Early pregnancy | Expectant and medical management of miscarriage |
| | Manual vacuum aspiration for miscarriage |
| | Expectant and medical management of ectopic pregnancy |

---

**Kim Lawson** MBChB, Clinical Research Fellow, Chelsea and Westminster Hospital, London, UK

**Cecilia Bottomley** MB BChir MRCOG MD, Consultant Obstetrician and Gynaecologist, Chelsea and Westminster Hospital, London, UK

(such as for management of a Bartholin's abscess) whereas in other conditions (such as outpatient management of hyperemesis) the patient may be seen daily for assessment and treatment in the ambulatory setting.

Early pregnancy units have, since the early 1990s led ambulatory care pathways in gynaecology, reducing hospital admissions by up to 40% [2]. Acute gynaecology units are a more recent development and may reduce hospital admissions by up to 48% [3].

In this chapter, we outline the common emergency gynaecology scenarios suited to ambulatory care and the principles and practicalities of this emerging care pathway.

## ACUTE GYNAECOLOGY

### Ambulatory management of hyperemesis gravidarum

#### Background

Severe nausea and vomiting of pregnancy (NVP) or hyperemesis gravidarum (HG) is one of the most common reasons for hospital admission in the first half of pregnancy with 0.3–3.6% [4] prevalence, and over 17,000 women in England requiring admission in 2010 [5].

Traditionally, a woman with NVP and ketonuria is admitted for inpatient rehydration and antiemetics, with an average length of stay of 3 days [5]. During this time a woman is away from her home, family and work, with physical, psychological and financial implications. Fiaschi et al. demonstrated that the prevalence of HG admissions and subsequent burden on hospitals has increased over time [5].

The ambulatory approach for management of HG allows women to attend on a daily basis for treatment, avoiding hospital admission in the majority of cases [6]. One randomised controlled trial (RCT) demonstrated a median two days hospital admission for women in the inpatient group compared with zero in the ambulatory group [7]. There was no difference in patient satisfaction and day care management was calculated to be 70% more cost effective compared to inpatient management. A further RCT showed no difference in eating, drinking, wellbeing or ketonuria at 48 hours and no difference in length of treatment or number of reattendances between women randomly assigned ambulatory versus inpatient care [8].

The Royal College of Obstetricians and Gynaecologists (RCOG) guideline (2016) recommends ambulatory care as first line for suitable women with NVP [9]. There is no evidence that initial symptom severity correlates with treatment efficacy, but the use of a severity score [Pregnancy-Unique Quantification of Emesis (PUQE)] is helpful to assess daily improvement [10]. More intensive inpatient support should be considered only for women with the following factors:

- Persistent nausea and vomiting despite regular oral antiemetics with weight loss >5% of body weight
- Medical comorbidities (e.g. diabetes, renal impairment, urinary tract infection)
- Serum potassium <3.2 mmol/L
- Serum sodium <130 mmol/L
- Third line treatment (steroid therapy) or parenteral nutrition required

#### Protocol for ambulatory management

After initial assessment for suitability for ambulatory care (as above) women should be assessed daily for symptom score, weight, ketonuria and electrolytes. At each daily

# Acute gynaecology

Table 7.2 Suggested protocol for ambulatory management of severe nausea and vomiting in pregnancy

| Daily observation and investigation | Daily treatment |
| --- | --- |
| Weight | Two 1L intravenous bags of 0.9% sodium chloride solution with 20 mmol of potassium chloride over a total of 4 hours |
| PUQE score | |
| BP, HR, temperature | Bolus antiemetic(s) either IV or IM on attendance (and ask to continue regular oral/buccal medication whilst at home between attendances) |
| Urinalysis for ketones | |
| Urea and electrolytes | Subcutaneous low molecular weight heparin prophylaxis (e.g. 40 mg enoxaparin) |
| | 1 pair Pabrinex ampoules weekly until tolerating tablets, then daily thiamine 50 mg and folic acid 5 mg |
| (Discharge from ambulatory care if 1+ or less ketones, able to tolerate food and no vomiting for 12 hours Admit if fits exclusion criteria listed) | |

attendance she receives rapid intravenous rehydration using normal saline with 20 mmol/L potassium chloride (maximum intravenous rate of 20 mmol potassium chloride per hour) and intramuscular or intravenous antiemetics. A first, second and third line antiemetic regime, vitamin replacement and thromboprophylaxis are all included in ambulatory management, as for inpatient care. A suggested protocol is in **Table 7.2**.

The treatment plan is discontinued when there is +1 or no ketonuria, the woman has not vomited for at least 12 hours and she has been able to tolerate some food and oral fluids. Women should be encouraged to continue with their antiemetic therapy once discharged until resolution of symptoms.

Given treatment for severe NVP is essentially supportive until spontaneous resolution, it is expected that, as for inpatient treatment, many women will have more than one treatment spell but specialist nurse-led telephone follow up may minimise reattendances or at least increase the number of days before further treatment is required by optimising outpatient care.

## Ambulatory management of Bartholin's cysts/abscesses

Bartholin's cysts or abscesses, developing when the distal portion of the duct from the Bartholin's gland is obstructed, affect around 2% of women, with abscesses being three times more common than cysts [11,12].

Definitive treatment options include:
- Traditional surgical incision, drainage and marsupialisation under general anaesthetic
- Insertion of an inflatable silicone or rubber balloon catheter after drainage under local anaesthetic

The inflatable balloon catheter (**Figure 7.1**) (also known as the word catheter) is simple to use and allows the drainage of the abscess followed by epithelialisation around the tube to induce fistula formation which allows the gland to continue to drain after subsequent removal of the catheter [12]. The technique is also suitable for other forms of vulval cyst and abscess.

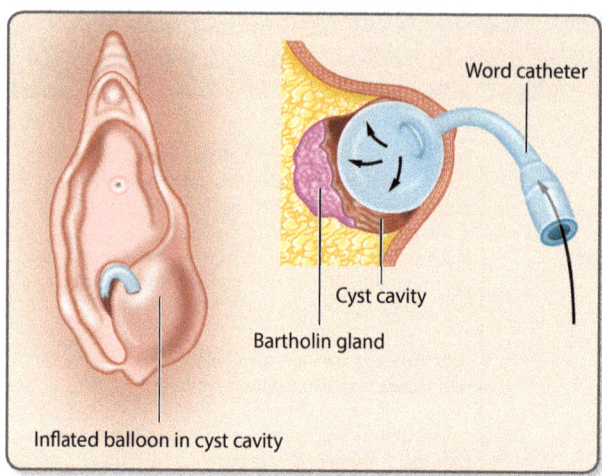

**Figure 7.1** Placement of Word catheter in a patient with a Bartholin gland cyst.

## Success rates

Reif et al. [13] showed an 87% success rate for initial placement of the catheter, with none of the 26 women having short-term recurrences. In another case series of 34 successful catheter insertions by Haider et al. [11] there was a 97% initial success rate with only one woman requiring marsupialisation due to recurrence of the abscess after the catheter fell out at 24 hours. Of those who had the catheter inserted for the full duration of treatment there were no recurrences by 6 months.

Kroese et al. [14] found patients reported increased pain at time of insertion of the balloon catheter but had fewer requirements for analgesia postprocedure when compared with marsupialisation.

In terms of time taken for the procedure, Boama et al. [15] demonstrated a significant impact on patient time saved, with a mean 40 minutes wait for the ambulatory procedure compared with 24 hours for patients admitted for the general anaesthetic procedure. Another study found an average of one hour to intervention for the catheter compared with 4 hours to marsupialisation [16]. The cost benefits extend to reduction in theatre time, theatre staff use and hospital admission costs [15]. The procedure is recognised as effective by the National Institute of Clinical Excellence (NICE) [12].

## Patient selection

Appropriate patient selection for the inflatable balloon catheter is important. Contraindications include: small cyst/abscess (size <3 cm is insufficient for balloon inflation), suspicion of malignancy (where examination under anaesthetic and possible biopsy should be considered) and a complex collection (as there is a perceived increased risk of failure if the cavity is too loculated) [12]. Recurrent abscess may still be suitable for a catheter depending on the degree of loculation.

## The procedure

In lithotomy position, the aseptic technique is adopted. Following local anaesthetic administration, a 3–5 mm stab incision is made into the medial aspect of the cyst or abscess (outside the hymenal ring) and the contents drained with gentle exploration of the cavity to ensure adequate drainage and breakdown of thin-walled septa. A pus sample is sent for culture if draining an abscess. The catheter is then inserted into the empty cavity (taking care not to insert it in between the vestibular mucosa and the cyst wall) and inflated with up to 3 mL saline (depending on the specific catheter manufacturer) to secure its position. The catheter is then left in situ for ideally 4 weeks.

Antibiotic treatment is not routine practice unless there is surrounding erythema/cellulitis or systemic symptoms.

Women should be reassured that they can return to normal daily activities (including exercise and sexual intercourse) after 3 days and for comfort the free end of the catheter can be tucked into the vagina. Little impingement on normal life is reported [16].

## Potential difficulties

A suture may be required to hold the balloon in place if the incision is too large. If the catheter falls out within 5 days of the initial procedure, reinsertion should be considered if the cavity is still identifiable. If a woman finds the catheter painful she should be seen again and have 1–2 mL of saline removed from the balloon to relieve the pressure.

## Hysteroscopic interventions in acute gynaecology

The use of the outpatient hysteroscopy is well established in the context of rapid access clinics for investigation of abnormal uterine bleeding [17]. However, practice in acute gynaecology units is less well established. Clinical conditions in the acute ambulatory gynaecology setting that might warrant hysteroscopic intervention include:
- Retrieval of an IUCD from within the uterine cavity
- Visualisation and removal of suspected retained tissue following miscarriage or termination
- Relief of pyometra or haematometra

A study of ambulatory hysteroscopic management of retained trophoblastic tissue, in women with average time to symptomatic presentation following termination of pregnancy of 35 days (range 2–105), found that the procedure was well tolerated and successful in 94.8% of cases [18]. Accurate confirmation of presence and location of the retained tissue is possible, minimising damage to the rest of the endometrial cavity (and risk of intrauterine adhesions) which can be associated with blind curettage. Hysteroscopic visualisation also allows for identification of any uterine anomalies that may be responsible for the retained tissue [18].

# EARLY PREGNANCY COMPLICATIONS

Ambulatory emergency gynaecology services, as an alternative to operating theatre procedures under general anaesthetic, include conservative management of miscarriage and ectopic pregnancy and manual vacuum aspiration (MVA) for miscarriage [19].

## Patient selection and advice

Managing expectations with ambulatory care for early pregnancy loss management is critical for the woman to feel confident and safe in her choice. Units offering outpatient management should provide 24-hour telephone access for advice and be able to arrange immediate hospital admission if required [19].

Women should be given an outline of the expected course of events, be advised of symptoms that warrant hospital attendance, and be offered appropriate analgesia and an aftercare plan. This is usually in the format of a repeat urine pregnancy test after 3 weeks[19]. A positive pregnancy test at 3 weeks or persistent bleeding after 2 weeks is signs of possible failure of treatment and indicates the need for reassesment with ultrasound scan.

## Outpatient management of miscarriage

### Expectant and medical management

As miscarriage is such a distressing event for women and their partners, the option of being in their own natural environment is a preferred choice for many. The NICE guideline recommends offering expectant management for the first 7–14 days to all suitable women following a diagnosis of miscarriage [19]. Medical management was initially limited to inpatient care but the majority of units now offer this as an ambulatory care pathway. However, there are subgroups of women for whom expectant or medical management is not recommended on clinical grounds (Table 7.3).

Vaginal misoprostol is the mainstay of medical treatment. The low reported incidence (1 in 70) of misoprostol-related complications, such as gastrointestinal side effects or heavy bleeding, supports its use in the outpatient setting [20]. Misoprostol dose and route of administration protocols for medical management of miscarriage vary and many units standardise protocols so that the same doses are given for incomplete and missed miscarriages. Current guidance does not recommend the routine use of mifepristone pretreatment in the management of first trimester miscarriage [19].

Success rates of medical management are higher in women diagnosed with incomplete miscarriage compared to those with a missed miscarriage (70–90% and 60–83% respectively) [21].

In some circumstances day admission to an ambulatory ward for medical management might be appropriate. Examples are advanced gestations, if tissue is needed for cytogenetic analysis or where there is an increased bleeding risk (such as twin gestation or possible coagulation disturbance). Prophylactic antibiotic cover may be given, however there is no increased risk of infection with either expectant or medical management when compared with surgical management (2–3% overall risk) [22].

**Table 7.3 Exclusion criteria for medical management of miscarriage**

Exclusion criteria
**Absolute**
- Allergy or contraindications to misoprostol +/- local anaesthetic agents

**Relative**
- Fetal demise >10 weeks' gestation
- Bleeding disorder
- Large fibroid uterus (>12/40 size or if suspected fibroids will affect access to uterine cavity)
- Evidence of infection
- Suspected molar pregnancy
- Known cervical stenosis
- Uterine malformations
- >4 cm retained products diagnosed on ultrasound, or if retained for more than 6 weeks (suspicion of calcification on ultrasound)
- Women who are unable to give informed consent

## Manual vacuum aspiration

The MVA carried out in the ambulatory setting is widely accepted as an alternative to surgical management of miscarriage [23]. The NICE guidance on the management of miscarriage recommends that women should be offered MVA if clinically appropriate [19]. However, the potential advantages and disadvantages mean it may not be suitable for all women (**Table 7.4**). The inclusion and exclusion criteria for MVA are summarised in **Table 7.5**.

The MVA was developed in the 1970s, and although subsequently superseded by electrical suction in the developed world, MVA has now been shown to be a preferable option for many women. The MVA technique applies the same principle as the conventional electrical suction but employs a single-use, handheld syringe [23]. The cannulas are latex-free, flexible and available in a range of sizes (4–12 mm).

An MVA may be carried out whenever surgical uterine evacuation may otherwise be recommended in early pregnancy. However in some cases, such as advanced gestation or high bleeding risk, it may be more appropriate to carry out a procedure under anaesthetic in theatre.

### Table 7.4 Suggested advantages and disadvantages of manual vacuum aspiration for miscarriage

| In favour | Against |
| --- | --- |
| Repeated high success rates in literature | Requires good communication during the procedure |
| High patient satisfaction levels | Distressing for some women due to awareness of evacuation |
| Less blood loss | Pain during the procedure |
| Theoretical reduced risk of uterine perforation | |
| Reduced waiting times for patients | |
| Significant cost savings compared to EVA | |

### Table 7.5 Inclusion and exclusion criteria for manual vacuum aspiration

**Inclusion criteria**
- Early fetal demise confirmed by ultrasound (<10 weeks' gestation)
- Ultrasound sac measurements of:
  - MSD ≤40 mm, CRL ≤25 mm or RPOC ≤4 cm
- Haemodynamically stable
- No clinical signs of infection
- Women who can easily tolerate speculum examination

**Exclusion criteria**
Absolute
- Allergy or contraindications to misoprostol +/− local anaesthetic agents

Relative
- Fetal demise >10 weeks' gestation
- Bleeding disorder
- Large fibroid uterus (>12/40 size or if suspected fibroids will affect access to uterine cavity)
- Evidence of infection
- Suspected molar pregnancy
- Known cervical stenosis
- Uterine malformations

## Procedure

Consent for the MVA under local anaesthetic should be carried out as for any surgical procedure. Patients should receive a detailed information leaflet and give informed written consent.

Cervical priming is recommended, especially in nulliparous patients with a diagnosis of missed miscarriage, to make dilatation of the cervix easier for the operator and less painful for the patient. Intravaginal misoprostol 400–800 µg, 1–3 hours prior to the procedure is a suggested regime, with concomitant simple analgesia [23]. An osmotic dilator can be used as an alternative, especially where misoprostol is contraindicated. The dilator should be inserted into the cervix 3–4 hours prior to the procedure.

The Cusco speculum is inserted and the cervix infiltrated with local anaesthetic (e.g. Prilocaine 3%, Citanest with Octapressin or 1% lidocaine). Once effective, the cannula and handheld suction device are used to gently evacuate the uterine cavity. The aspirated contents should be visualised to confirm products of conception and sent for histological examination if required. The signs suggesting completion of evacuation of the uterus are noting red or pink foam without tissue passing through the cannula, a 'gritty' sensation as the cannula passes over the surface of the evacuated uterine cavity and the uterus contracting around the cannula. The woman should be warned that she may feel increased cramping towards the end of the procedure, when the uterus is empty and contracting.

## Ultrasound

There is no evidence base for MVA to be carried out under ultrasound control. However, in the authors' experience, performing MVA in an outpatient procedure room with transvaginal ultrasound available, there is some advantage to confirming the absence of significant retained tissue at the end of the procedure, though absence of ultrasound is not a contraindication to the procedure.

Following completion of the MVA, an IUCD can be safely inserted if required. The patient should then be allowed to recover in a comfortable area, closely monitored by nursing staff for 1–2 hours.

## Success rates

Reported success rates for MVA are more than 95% [23]. The nature of complications after manual aspiration is the same as expected after electrical suction curettage (haemorrhage, uterine perforation, incomplete evacuation leading to repeat aspiration, cervical laceration). Importantly the rate of intrauterine adhesions may be lower than with electrical suction under general anaesthesia [24].

## Ambulatory management of ectopic pregnancy

Ambulatory medical or expectant management is suitable for many women with a tubal ectopic pregnancy or with a medically managed non-tubal ectopic pregnancy [25]. Additionally, as ectopic pregnancies are commonly diagnosed early with high resolution transvaginal ultrasound, day unit admission for surgical management is suitable for women with small asymptomatic tubal ectopic pregnancies and some stable nontubal ectopic pregnancies, such as caesarean scar pregnancies.

To allow continuity and ease-of-access for patients, follow-up should be managed from a single point of care (whether early pregnancy unit or ambulatory care unit). Robust

| Table 7.6 Inclusion criteria for expectant and medical management of ectopic pregnancy | |
|---|---|
| **Expectant management** | **Medical management** |
| Asymptomatic | Asymptomatic |
| Haemodynamically stable | Haemodynamically stable |
| Initial hCG <1500 units/L | Initial hCG <5000 units/L |
| No evidence of intrauterine pregnancy or significant haemoperitoneum on US | A confirmed ectopic pregnancy without fetal cardiac activity or significant haemoperitoneum on US |
| No tenderness on bimanual examination or TVUS | No significant tenderness on bimanual or abdominal examination |
| Able to comply with follow-up | Able to comply with follow-up |
| | Ectopic mass <35 mm in all single diameters |
| | No contraindications to methotrexate: renal or liver impairment, breastfeeding, immunodeficiency, active peptic ulcer |

pathways for referral from the emergency department and for acute admissions during out-of-hours should be in place. Ambulatory management is not appropriate if a unit is unable to provide 24-hour telephone support or if patients are deemed unlikely to be compliant with the strict follow-up required [2].

Up to 50% of women diagnosed with an ectopic pregnancy may be suitable for expectant management and success rates, although dependent upon the inclusion criteria, may be up to 70% [26,27]. In suitable women **(Table 7.6)** who opt for expectant management approximately 30% ultimately require intervention (usually surgical) because of rising human chorionic gonadotropin (hCG) levels or due to development of symptoms [27].

Medical management (with methotrexate) success rates vary from 65–95% [26]. Predictors of success are the similar to those predicting expectant management (empty/absent gestation sac and increased time from LMP) and lower rise in hCG prior to commencing treatment [25].

In light of the cytotoxic properties of methotrexate and the occasional false positive ultrasound diagnosis of ectopic pregnancy, it is critical that there is no possibility of an ongoing intrauterine pregnancy prior to methotrexate administration [28].

## Patient selection and advice

All appropriate treatment options should be discussed with a patient and contacts given for support groups provided such as Ectopic Pregnancy Trust in the UK [25]. The risks and benefits of each modality need to be addressed and the patient's choice taken into consideration.

Detailed written information for medical management of ectopic pregnancy should be provided about the possible side effects of methotrexate and the following recommendations should be given [19]:
- Maintain good hydration, avoid alcohol, avoid folic acid and vitamin supplements and avoid sexual intercourse until hCG levels are within normal limits
- Avoid direct exposure to sunlight for 1 week following treatment

- Avoid nonsteroidal antiinflammatory medication for 1 week after treatment
- Delay conception for 3 months after treatment (teratogenic effects of methotrexate)

**Follow-up for ambulatory management of ectopic pregnancy**

Women with expectant or medically managed ectopic pregnancy should undergo continuous follow-up until they meet criteria for discharge from care (hCG <5 IU/L and asymptomatic).

## EFFECTIVE RUNNING OF AN AMBULATORY GYNAECOLOGY UNIT

### Development of the service

With rising emergency department attendances, ambulatory emergency care in gynaecology is increasingly recognised as an essential new approach requiring redesign of systems as part of the solution to manage demand for hospital resources. Ambulatory care can have a similar impact on emergency care as day surgery has had on planned care. However for emergency patients presenting to hospital for admission to be rapidly assessed, streamed to ambulatory care and diagnosed and treated, processes need to be in place, including review by a consultant and timely access to diagnostics and treatments, all delivered within one working day [29,30].

The concept of experience-based design involves looking at the care journey and in addition the emotional journey people experience when they come into contact with a particular pathway or part of the service. The traditional view of the user as a passive recipient of a product or service is replaced by the view of users as integral to the improvement and innovation process. In ambulatory emergency gynaecology with significant emotional effects of most conditions treated, this design process is especially relevant with multiple tools available to implement effective care [31].

### Procedures

Despite the procedures described, such as MVA and balloon catheter insertion for the Bartholin's abscess occurring in an ambulatory procedure room rather than an operating theatre, the same principles of surgical safety apply. In particular, appropriate informed consent and a World Health Organisation (WHO) style safety checklist should be completed [32].

Women require a calm and secure environment when undertaking gynaecology procedures and consideration needs to be given to this environment. As the patient is awake (and non-sedated) during the procedure, particular care and attention should be made to maintaining and respecting the patient's dignity throughout. Planning of the acute gynaecology procedural room includes availability of music, supportive nursing or health care assistants, chaperones, lockable doors and appropriate lighting, all of which contribute to the patient experience.

### Staffing

For an ambulatory unit to be efficient and effective, it requires a multidisciplinary approach. The majority of units are run by specialist-trained nurses, many of whom have additional ultrasound scanning and procedural skills (e.g. MVA or Bartholin's abscess drainage). Otherwise, sonographers or medical staff will perform ultrasound which is generally the pivotal diagnostic tool in ambulatory acute gynaecology care.

## Multidisciplinary meetings

Multidisciplinary discussion of complex and challenging cases in ambulatory care is essential for appropriate clinical decision-making and shared learning, as in other subspecialties in Obstetrics and Gynaecology. Governance requirements mandate risk events should be reported regularly to the multidisciplinary team. Multidisciplinary groups are as in other areas of medicine, effective conduits for the defining and achieving the required standards in emergency gynaecology [33].

## Patient access

To prevent hospital admission, timely access to an ambulatory acute gynaecology unit is important. Therefore, in setting up a unit the pathways from general practitioners and emergency departments should aim to minimise the time from first referral to diagnosis and definitive management. Pathways will be dependent on local situations but specific telephone or electronic referral with timely response is imperative.

> **Key points for clinical practice**
>
> - All gynaecology departments should be developing ambulatory care units for women with acute gynaecology and early pregnancy problems, as the reduction in hospital admissions as a result is estimated at 40%.
> - The MVA should be offered to all eligible women as part of the counselling for miscarriage management.
> - Insertion of an inflatable balloon catheter following incision and drainage of a Bartholin's cyst or abscess under local anaesthetic has equivalent results to traditional marsupialisation with significant patient and healthcare cost benefits.
> - Ambulatory management of hyperemesis daily as an outpatient is equivalent in efficacy to traditional inpatient management, with the advantage of maintaining social function for the woman and decreased cost to the healthcare provider.
> - Ectopic pregnancy and miscarriage can frequently be managed expectantly, medically or surgically without hospital admission provided close ambulatory care monitoring is available.
> - Ambulatory acute gynaecology units benefit from the same multidisciplinary discussion forums and governance procedures as other specialties.
> - Staff and user experiences are critical in development of modern services for ambulatory care in emergency gynaecology.

## REFERENCES

1. Ambulatory Emergecy Care Network. Available from: http://www.ambulatoryemergencycare.org.uk. / Tools-and-Resources/Experience-Based-Design-EBD. [Accessed 1 April 2017]
2. Jones K, Pearce C. Organising an acute gynaecology service: equipment, setup and a brief review of the likely conditions that are managed in the unit. Best Pract Res CLin Obstet Gynaecol 2009; 4:427–438.

3. Haider Z, Condous G, Khalid A, et al. The impact of the availability of ultrasonography on the acute gynaecology unit. Ultrasound Obstet Gynceol 2006; 28:207–213.
4. Einarson TR, Piwko C, Koren G. Quantifying the global rates of nausea and vomiting of pregnancy: a meta analysis. 2013; 20:e171–183.
5. Fiaschi L, Nelson-Piercy C, Tata LJ. Hospital admission for hyperemesis gravidarum: a nationwide study of occurrence, reoccurrence and risk factors among 8.2 million pregnancies. Hum Reprod 2016; 31:1675–1684.
6. McCarthy FP, Lutomski JE, Greene RA. Hyperemesis gravidarum: current persepctives. Int J Womens Health 2014; 6:719–725.
7. Murphy A, McCarthy FP, McElroy B, et al. Day care versus inpatient management of nausea and vomiting of pregnancy: cost utility analysis of a randomised controlled trial. Eur J Obstet Gynecol Reprod Biol 2016; 197:78–82.
8. Mitchell-Jones N, Farren JA, Tobias A, et al. Ambulatory versus inpatient management of severe nausea and vomiting of pregnancy: a randomised control trial with patient preference arm. BMJ Open. 2017; 7:e017566.
9. Royal College of Obstetricians and Gynaecologists. The Management of Nausea and Vomiting of Pregnancy and Hyperemesis Gravidarum. RCOG Greentop Guideline No 69. London. June 2016.
10. Haider Z, Condous G, Kirk E, et al. The simple outpatient management of Bartholin's abscess using the Word catheter: A preliminary study. Aust N Z J Obstet Gynaecol. 2007; 47:137–140.
11. Haider Z, Condous G, Kirk E, et al. The simple outpatient management of Bartholin's abscess using the Word catheter: A preliminary study. Aust N Z J Obstet Gynaecol. 2007; 47:137 -140.
12. National Institute for Health and Clinical Excellence. Balloon catheter insertion for Bartholin's cyst or abscess. Interventional procedures guidance [IPG323], 2009.
13. Reif P, Ulrich D, Bjelic-Radisic V, et al. Management of Bartholin's cyst and abscess using the Word catheter: implementation, recurrence rates and costs. Eur J Obstet Gynecol Reprod Biol 2015; 190:81–84.
14. Kroese JA, van der Velde M, Morssink LP, et al. Word catheter and marsupialisation in women with a cyst or abscess of the Bartholin gland (WoMan-trial): a randomised clinical trial. BJOG 2017; 124:243–249.
15. Boama V, Horton J. Word balloon catheter for Bartholin's cyst and abscess as an office procedure: clinical time gained. BMC Research Notes 2016; 9:13.
16. Reif P, Elsayed H, Ulrich D, et al. Quality of life and sexual activity during treatment of Bartholin's cyst or abscess with a Word catheter. Eur J Obstet Gynecol Reprod Biol 2015; 190:76–80.
17. Royal College of Obstetricians and Gynaecologists. Clinical green top guidelines. Best practice in outpatient hysteroscopy. London: RCOG Press, March 2011.
18. Jimenez J, Gonzales C, Alvarez C, et al. Conservative management of retained trophoblastic tissue and placental polyp with diagnostic ambulatory hysteroscopy. Eur J Obstet Gynecol Reprod Biol 2009; 145:89–92.
19. National Institute for Health and Care Excellence. Ectopic Pregnancy and Miscarriage: Diagnosis and Initial Management in Early Pregnancy of Ectopic Pregnancy and Miscarriage. NICE Clinical Guideline 154. London: NICE; 2012.
20. Zhang J, Gilles JM, et al. A comparison of medical management with misoprostol and surgical management for early pregnancy failure. N Eng J Med 2005; 353:761–769.
21. Graziosi GC, Mol BW, et al. management of early pregnancy loss. Int J Gynaecol Obstet 2004; 86:337-46
22. Trinder J, Brocklehurst P, Porter R, et al. Management of miscarriage: expectant, medical or surgical? Results of randomsied controlled trial (miscarriage treatment (MIST) trial). BMJ 2006; 332:1235.
23. Sharma M. Manual vacuum aspiration: an outpatient alternative for surgical management of miscarriage. Obstet Gynaecol 2015; 17:157–61.
24. Gilman AR, Dewar KM, Rhone SA, Fluker MR. Intrauterine Adhesions Following Miscarriage: Look and Learn. J Obstet Gynaecol Can 2016; 38:453–457.
25. Royal College of Obstetricians and Gynaecologists. Diagnosis and Management of Ectopic Pregnancy. RCOG Green-top guideline No. 21; Joint with the Association of Early Pregnancy Units. London. November 2016.
26. Kirk EJ, Condous G, et al. The non-surgical management of ectopic pregnancy. Ultrasound Obstet Gynecol 2006; 27:91–100.
27. Mavrelos D, Nicks H, Jamil, A, et al. Efficacy and safety of a clinical protocol for expectant management of selected women diagnosed with a tubal ectopic pregnancy. Ultrasound Obstet Gynecol 2013; 42:102–107.
28. Kirk E, Bottomley C, Bourne T. Diagnosing ectopic pregnancy and current concepts in the management of pregnancy of unknown location. Hum Reprod Update 2014; 20:250–261.

29. Royal College of Physicians. Acute care toolkit 10: ambulatory emergency care. London:RCP, 2014. https://www.rcplondon.ac.uk/guidelines-policy/acute-care-toolkit-10-ambulatory-emergency-care [Accessed 1 April 2017]
30. Ambulatory Emergency Care Network. NHS Elect. Directory of Ambulatory Emergency Care for Adults. http://www.ambulatoryemergencycare.org.uk/Tools-and-Resources/AEC-Directory [Accessed 1 April 2017]
31. NHS Elect. Experience based design guide. http://www.ambulatoryemergencycare.org.uk/Tools-and-Resources/Experience-Based-Design-EBD [Accessed 1 April 2017]
32. WHO Surgical Safety Checklist. http://www.who.int/patientsafety/safesurgery/checklist/en/Checklist [Accessed 1 April 2017]
33. Royal College of Obstetricians and Gynaecologists. Gynaecology Standards. London. Guidelines and reports, 2016.

# Chapter 8

## Hereditary cancer in gynaecology: What clinicians should know about genetic-testing, screening and risk reduction

*Faiza Maryam Gaba, Ranjit Manchanda*

## INTRODUCTION

The field of cancer genetics has seen an exponential growth in recent years leading to an increased interest, focus and awareness on management of hereditary cancers. Ovarian and endometrial cancers have a significant genetic component. Twin studies suggest that 22% of ovarian cancer (OC) risk can be explained by inheritable factors [1]. *BRCA1/BRCA2* mutations account for most of the known inheritable risk of OC and are found in around 10-18% of non-mucinous high grade epithelial OC cases [2 3]. Nevertheless, *BRCA1/BRCA2* mutations explain only 1/4th of the familial relative risk for OC [4 5]. Around 3% (1.6-5.9%) patients with endometrial cancer (EC) [6-9] and ~1% epithelial-OC cases [3,10,11] have mismatch repair (*MMR*) gene (*MLH1/MSH2/MSH6/PMS2*) mutations or Lynch syndrome (LS). Traditionally, hereditary gynaecological cancers have been broadly categorised within three main syndromes associated with autosomal dominant gene mutations:

- Hereditary breast and ovarian cancer (HBOC): families with multiple cases of breast and ovarian cancer
- Hereditary ovarian cancer (HOC): families with multiple cases of ovarian cancer only; and
- Lynch syndrome: The tumour spectrum comprises a number of cancers of which colorectal cancer (CRC), EC, and OC are the commonest [12-14]. Additionally, it includes gastric, small bowel, hepatobiliary, brain, ureteric and renal pelvic (upper urologic tract) cancers. LS is caused by a mutation in one of the *MMR* genes.

---

**Faiza Maryam Gaba** MBBS, MRCOG Clinical Research Fellow in Gynaecological Oncology, Barts Cancer Institute, Queen Mary University of London, London, UK.

**Ranjit Manchanda** MD, MRCOG, PhD Clinical Senior Lecturer, Consultant Gynaecological Oncologist Barts Cancer Institute, Queen Mary University of London, London, UK.

|  | Hereditary breast and ovarian cancer | Hereditary ovarian cancer | Lynch syndrome | Cowden's syndrome | Peutz–Jeghers syndrome |
|---|---|---|---|---|---|
| Gene Mutations | BRCA1, BRCA2 | BRCA1, BRCA2, RAD51C, RAD51D, BRIP1 | MMR (MLH1/MSH2/MSH6/PMS2/EPCAM) | PTEN | STK11/LKB1 |
| Ovary | ✓ | ✓ | ✓ |  |  |
| Breast | ✓ |  |  |  |  |
| Endometrium |  | ✓ | ✓ | ✓ |  |
| Cervix |  | ✓ |  |  | ✓ |
| Other |  |  | Colon, gastric, ureteral, biliary, pancreatic, glioblastoma | Colon, thyroid, benign hamartomas | Bowel hamartomas, gastric, pancreatic |

Table 8.1 Syndromes in hereditary gynaecological cancer

The gynaecological cancer syndromes and associated gene mutations are listed in Table 8.1.

## MUTATIONS AND CANCER RISK

### BRCA1/BRCA2 mutations

Around 1 in 300 individuals in the general population carry a *BRCA1/BRCA2* gene mutation. These mutations occur more frequently in certain founder populations such as the Ashkenazi Jewish (AJ) population, 1 in 40 of whom carry one of three common *BRCA1/BRCA2* Jewish founder mutations [15]. Founder mutations have also been reported in other populations: Icelandic, Polish, Norwegian, etc [16]. *BRCA1* carriers have a 44% risk of OC, 71% risk of BC till 80 years age. *BRCA2* carriers have a 17% OC-risk and 69% BC-risk till 80 years [17]. *BRCA2* men also have a 7% risk of BC and 18–25% risk of prostate cancer [18 19]. *BRCA1* men have only a small increase in prostate cancer risk. There is also an increased risk of pancreatic cancer associated mainly with the *BRCA2* gene (~5% risk) [20].

### RAD51C, RAD51D and BRIP1 gene mutations:

*RAD51C, RAD51D* and *BRIP1* are newer moderate penetrance OC genes, whose risks were recently validated. The OC-risk with *RAD51C* or *RAD51D* is around 11% and with BRIP1 is ~6% [21-23]. These genes are not associated with an increased risk of BC.

### MMR gene mutations:

*MMR* genes include *MLH1, MSH2, MSH6* and *PMS2. MMR* gene mutations cause LS. The Amsterdam criteria-II (AC-II) have been traditionally used to identify LS [24]. AC- II criteria include:
- At least three relatives in the family with one of the LS cancers (described above), all of whom should be related by a first degree relationship to each other
- LS cancers should span at least two generations, and
- At least one of the LS cancers should be <50 years [24]. This is also called the 3:2:1 rule. MMR mutations are associated with 40–60% risk of CRC, 30–60% risk of EC and around 10% (6–14%) risk of OC [14].

### *PTEN* gene mutations

*PTEN* gene mutations cause an autosomal dominant condition called Cowden's syndrome. These mutations are associated with a 10–28% risk of EC. [25,26], but OC risk is not increased. It is also associated with a 50% risk of BC and 3–10% risk of thyroid cancer.

### *STK11 (LKB1)* gene mutations

*STK11/LKB1* mutations cause Peutz–Jeghers syndrome (PJS). It is characterised by polyps throughout the gastrointestinal tract and mucocutaneous pigmentation. PJS is associated with an increased risk of a rare cervical cancer called adenoma malignum. While EC and OC cases have been reported in some series, it is predominantly associated with benign sex cord stromal ovarian tumours [27,28]. It is also associated with an increased risk of breast and gastrointestinal cancers.

## GENETIC-TESTING AND RISK ASCERTAINMENT

### Family history or clinical criteria based assessment

A family history (FH) or pedigree based assessment involves a detailed evaluation of cancer history in the patient and across three generations of the family. This should include both maternal and paternal sides of the family (affected and unaffected relatives), ethnicity, age of family members, age of cancer onset, histological details, age of death, genetic-testing undertaken with the test result, any known mutation in the family. Details/results of any molecular testing undertaken on tumour tissue; and prophylactic or relevant surgical history should also be documented. This information is then used to assess the probability of the presence of a known gene mutation in the family.

Over the years a number of risk models and/or clinical criteria have been used to identify and categorise families as high-risk. Genetic-testing has then be offered to individuals fulfilling these criteria or those exceeding predefined mutation carrier probability thresholds predicted by using these models or risk criteria. Models vary widely depending on the population characteristics/datasets and the statistical methodology used, the extent and detail of family cancer history incorporated, various risk factors included/excluded and underlying assumptions. They are broadly classified into Empirical and Mendelian models. Empirical models use variables describing FH to discriminate between positive and negative families, usually using logistic regression. They are more straightforward to use/implement and readily incorporate nongenetic risk factors. A widely used example is the Manchester scoring system (MSS) [29]. Mendelian models can deal better with complex family histories. They incorporate the allele frequency of susceptibility genes in the population and penetrance estimates for these alleles in carriers and noncarriers. Pedigree based analysis with Mendelian rules of genetic transmission and Bayesian calculations are used to develop a genetic model for disease. Widely used examples include BOADICEA (Cambridge, UK) [30] and BRCAPRO (Bayes-Mendel, USA) [31] and Tyrer-Cuzick (London, UK). These models provide individualised probabilities of risk or carrying a mutation.

The National Institute for Health and Care Excellence (NICE) recommends *BRCA1/BRCA2* testing be offered to those who have a 10% combined *BRCA1/BRCA2* probability [32]. This threshold of offering genetic-testing in the UK was previously 20% and became 10% in 2013. Commonly used risk models in the UK are MSS and BOADICEA. MSS cannot account for AJ families and is not suitable for them. MSS (MSS-3) scores of 15 and

20 correspond to a 10% and 20% *BRCA1+BRCA2* carrier probabilities respectively [29]. Looser clinical-criteria are in use for AJ families given the higher *BRCA* prevalence in this population. **Table 8.2** provides easy to read and use clinical-criteria used for identifying high-risk individuals in the London Cancer Familial Gynaecological Cancer MDT (Barts Health NHS Trust, University College London Hospital).

The customary FH approach to genetic-testing has involved testing affected individuals from high-risk families via high-risk cancer genetic clinics after face-to-face pre-test genetic counselling by geneticists/genetic counsellors. For this to be effective, it is important for individuals and their doctors to recognise significant FH and act on it. However, a number of mutation carriers are unaware of their FH or its significance, are not proactive in seeking advice, or may well lack a strong enough FH and thus get excluded from the process. FH based prediction models are only moderately effective at predicting the presence of *BRCA1/BRCA2* mutations and have poor negative likelihood ratios or poor ability for predicting the absence of one [33]. Around 50% mutation carriers lack a strong FH and are not identified by FH-based testing [15-34-36].

## Lynch syndrome

The AC-II described above, have been traditionally used to identify LS [24]. However, the AC-II criteria alone miss 55–70% of mutation carriers. [6,37,38] Hence, laxer criteria called the Revised Bethesda-criteria [39] were introduced to improve ascertainment by identifying CRC cases for molecular analysis (immunohistochemistry (IHC) and/or Microsatellite-instability (MSI)) as an initial step. Genetic-testing is subsequently undertaken for IHC protein deficient or MSI unstable tumours [24]. Bethesda-criteria too can miss 12-30% of MMR carriers [40]. IHC/MSI analysis for all EC and CRC cases is better at identifying MMR carriers than AC-II/Bethesda/modified age linked criteria alone [37,41-43]. Hence, IHC/MSI testing for all CRC cases is now recommended and is gradually being implemented. IHC/MSI testing for EC cases has recently been recommended but practice varies with centers offering testing in cases <50 or <60 or at all ages. Implementation is patchy and this is not yet common practice in the UK, but is likely to change in the future.

## Testing of unselected cancer case series

The availability of next generation sequencing (NGS) technologies, falling costs coupled with loosening of the threshold/criteria for genetic-testing, and increasing availability of options for targeted precision medicine driven treatment, have led to the promotion and propagation of unselected cancer case series testing, with genetic-testing offered at cancer diagnosis. NICE (UK) [32] and other international guidelines [44-46] recommend *BRCA1/BRCA2*-testing be offered at ≥10% carrier probability, making women with high grade non-mucinous epithelial-OC (BRCA-prevalence 10–18%) [2,3,47] or triple negative BC (BRCA-prevalence ~10%) [48,49] eligible for genetic-testing. Hence, NHS-England [50] and other guidelines [46] now recommend *BRCA*-testing for all non-mucinous EOC and triple negative BC, and many centres in North America and Europe have adopted this practice.

Reflex testing (IHC/MSI) of tumour tissue in all CRC and more recently all EC has been advocated to increase ascertainment for LS. Genetic-testing is then recommended for those individuals whose tumour tissue stains negative for the MMR protein on IHC or whose tumour tissue shows an unstable MSI result. Informed pre-test counselling is undertaken before genetic-testing.

### Table 8.2 Criteria to identify high risk families (London Cancer MDT) [121-126]

Volunteer/proband should either have been affected by cancer or be a FDR of an affected family member. Affected relatives should be on the same side of the family (i.e. maternal or paternal)

**Families with ovarian\* or ovarian\* and breast cancer**
- \>2 individuals with ovarian cancer (any age) who are first degree relatives (FDR)
- 1 ovarian cancer (any age) and 1 breast cancer <50 who are FDR
- 1 ovarian cancer (any age) and 2 breast cancers <60 who are FDR
- Breast cancer in volunteer/ proband and FDR with both breast and ovarian cancer (in the same person)
- Woman with both breast and ovarian cancer (in the same person)
- Criteria 1, 2 and 3 can be modified where paternal transmission is occurring, i.e. families where affected relatives are related by second through an unaffected intervening male relative and there is an affected sister eligible

\* History of tubal/primary peritoneal cancers may be considered equivalent to ovarian cancer.

**Families with a known gene mutation**
The family contains an affected individual with a mutation in 1 of the known ovarian/endometrial cancer predisposing genes, e.g. BRCA1, BRCA2, RAD51C, RAD51D, BRIP1, MLH1, MSH2, MSH6, PMS2, PTEN, STK11/LKB1

**Lynch syndrome/HNPCC families**
- The family contains three or more individuals with a LS or HNPCC related cancer\*, who are FDR and >1 case is diagnosed before 50 years and the cancers affect >1 generation
- Molecular (IHC/MSI) analysis of unselected colorectal cases and unselected endometrial cancer cases is recommended to identify those who can have MMR gene testing\*\*

\*LS or HNPCC related cancers include: colorectal, endometrial, ovarian, small bowel, ureteric, hepatobiliary, brain and renal pelvic cancers.
\*\*While this is recommended, practice varies with centers offering testing in cases under 50 or under 60 or at all ages. Unselected testing irrespective of age is now recommended.

**Families with only breast cancer**
- 4 breast cancers in the family (any ages)
- 3 breast cancers related by FDR:
  - 1 <30 years or
  - 2 <40 years or
  - All <60 years or
  - 1 male breast cancer (MBC) and 2 breast cancers <60 years
- Breast cancer in volunteer/proband (<50 years):
  - Breast cancer in mother (age of onset being <30 years) or
  - Bilateral breast cancer in mother (<40 years onset) or
  - 1 FDR with MBC
- 2 MBC in the family and proband is a FDR of 1 of them

**Families with Ashkenazi Jewish (AJ) or Polish ancestry\***
- Female breast cancer diagnosed <50
- FDR with female breast cancer diagnosed <50
- Male BRCA-related cancer (breast/prostate /pancreas) any age
- FDR with male breast cancer

\*BRCA Founder mutation testing only

**Women with non-mucinous invasive high grade epithelial ovarian cancer (EOC)**
- Women (any age) with invasive non mucinous high grade EOC regardless of family history/ethnicity.

**Women with triple negative (TN) breast cancer**
- Women with TN breast cancer (any age)

**Manchester Scoring System (MSS)**
- Manchester score ≥15

**BOADICEA/BRCAPRO**
- Combined BRCA1 & BRCA2 probability ≥10% using one of the above risk models

EOC, epithelial ovarian cancer; FDR, first degree relative; IHC, immunohistochemistry; LS, Lynch syndrome; HNPCC, Hereditary non-polyposis colorectal cancer; MBC, male breast cancer; MSI, microsatellite instability; TN, triple negative

## Panel testing

The NGS has enabled simultaneous testing of multiple genes (panel-testing) with high throughput. Many newer moderate penetrance genes have been discovered over the last few years as a result of which panel-testing for multiple genes is becoming common practice. However, a number of commercially driven panels offer genetic-testing for a large number of genes, a number of whose risks have not been properly validated and therefore lack clinical utility. This is a matter of significant concern. It is important that clinical-testing be undertaken for genes with well-defined 'clinical utility' and testing for other genes be restricted to the research setting.

## Informed counselling and genetic-testing

Eligible at-risk women identified should be offered informed pre-test counselling and genetic-testing. Informed consent prior to testing should include pre-test education and counselling covering the risks, benefits and limitations of testing, the implications of positive and negative test results as well as variants of uncertain significance. Clinicians/health professionals performing genetic-testing should have adequate training, expertise and knowledge to be able to effectively counsel patients.

Different models of pre-test counselling have evolved over the years. The traditional approach involved face-to-face counselling by the genetics clinician/genetic counsellor in a specialist genetics clinic. Randomised trial data show that telephone counselling as well as use of decision-aids and DVD-based counselling are equally effective [51-53]. With the advent of cancer case series testing and need for large scale implementation, counselling has now moved into the realm of non-genetics clinicians. Under the mainstreaming model counselling and genetic-testing at cancer diagnosis is undertaken by the medical oncologist and coordinated by the genetics service [2]. Under the cancer MDT coordinated precision medicine (CMP) model, all nongenetics clinicians (surgeons, medical oncologists and clinical oncologists) undertake counselling and genetic-testing and this is coordinated through the gynaecological cancer MDT [54]. Test results are given to the patient by the clinician performing testing. Individuals with positive results are subsequently referred to the genetics service for further management and undertaking predictive testing in the family. Nongenetics clinicians undertake counselling after adequate training, including on line modules and didactic teaching.

As testing costs fall further in the future, germline-sequencing could eventually potentially become the first line test for EC, obviating the need for MSI/IHC triage. The applicability of genomics in medicine and incorporation into routine care is increasing. It will eventually become essential for all gynaecologists to be trained in undertaking counselling for genetic-testing and understanding its implications.

## Advantages of genetic-testing

In women diagnosed with epithelial-OC, it offers the opportunity for targeted treatment. Maintenance Olaparib in *BRCA1/BRCA2* mutated platinum sensitive relapsed epithelial-OC significantly improves progression free survival (HR = 0.18, 95% CI:0·10–0·31) [55] and overall survival (HR = 0·73, 95% CI:0·55–0·96) [55,56]. This benefit was found in patients with germline and/or somatic mutations. Thus Olaparib/PARP inhibitor has recently been approved by the European Commission, the US Food and Drug Administration (FDA) and NICE for patients with recurrent *BRCA*-mutated ovarian, fallopian or peritoneal cancer [57-59]. In addition family members of patients found to carry a pathogenic germline mutation can be offered predictive testing. Unaffected at-risk mutation carriers have a number of options to minimise or reduce their OC and BC risk. They can opt for: risk-reducing salpingo-oophorectomy (RRSO) to reduce their OC-risk [60,61]; MRI/mammography screening, risk-reducing mastectomy (RRM) [62], or chemoprevention with selective estrogen-receptor-modulators (SERM) to reduce their BC-risk [63]; better lifestyle/reproductive choices, as well as pre-implantation genetic-diagnosis (PGD) [64].

Effective interventions for preventing CRC, EC and OC exist for LS women too. LS/MMR carriers can opt for prophylactic hysterectomy and bilateral salpingo-oophoprectomy to prevent EC and OC. They can also benefit from 1–2 yearly colonoscopies for CRC screening and daily aspirin [65-67] to reduce CRC risk [41].

### Disadvantages of genetic-testing

Risks include potential impact on psychological health. Some individuals may feel distressed about positive results and guilty about passing mutations to their children. Given familial implications it could also affect family dynamics and relationships. Other issues to consider are marriage-ability (relevant for some communities) and potential implications for insurance/employment. In the US, the GINA (Genetic-Information Non-discrimination Act) and in the UK a moratorium between Department of Health and Association of British Insurers provide a level of protection against using test results for setting insurance premiums.

### Population-based genetic-testing

The limitations of FH or clinical-criteria based testing can be overcome by population-based testing, i.e. offering genetic-testing to an entire population irrespective of any FH of cancer. NGS technologies with high-throughput multiplex panel testing, falling costs and advances in computational bioinformatics has made population-testing technically feasible. Population-based testing for *BRCA1/BRCA2* genes has been extensively investigated in the AJ population, through a UK randomised controlled trial (RCT) (GCaPPS: Genetic Cancer Prediction through Population Screening) and two cohort studies (in Israel, Canada) [15,34,68]. RCT data show that population-based BRCA-testing in AJ is acceptable, does not detrimentally affect psychological well-being or quality of life, can be undertaken in a community setting, identifies more mutation carriers, and is extremely cost-effective [15,52,69]. Unselected BRCA-testing in the AJ-population fulfils the principles of population-based genetic-testing [70]. There is good evidence to support change in practice and implementation of population-based BRCA-testing in the AJ-population and a number of scientists have advocated this. However, results from the AJ-population cannot be directly extrapolated to the general non-Jewish population and further research into population-testing is required in the general population. A pilot feasibility study (PROMISE-FS) is ongoing in the UK [71].

## GYNAECOLOGICAL CANCER SCREENING IN HIGH RISK WOMEN

### Ovarian cancer screening

Following evidence of survival benefit, [72] three RCTs investigated OC-screening in low-risk postmenopausal women: Japanese Shizuoka [73]; USA PLCO (Prostate Lung Colorectal and Ovarian) cancer screening [74] and the UKCTOCS (United Kingdom Collaborative Trial on Ovarian Cancer Screening) trials. The first two used annual ultrasound and absolute CA125 value for OC-screening. The Japanese trial ($n$ = 82,400) reported a statistically non-significant higher proportion of stage-I OC with screening (63%) compared to controls (38%) [73]. The PLCO and UKCTOCS trials evaluated the mortality impact of OC-screening. The PLCO trial ($n$ = 78,216) reported no mortality benefit, only 28% early stage I/II OC and a high 15% complication rate from diagnostic bilateral salpingo-oophorectomy (BSO) [75]. The UKCTOCS study ($n$ = 202,000) differed significantly from the Shizuoka/PLCO trails as it investigated a sequential longitudinal CA125 biomarker based screening strategy using ROCA (risk of ovarian cancer algorithm) along with an annual ultrasound based screening strategy in a 1:1:2 randomised design. The results of the ROCA driven multimodal screening strategy appear especially promising. ROCA-based screening has a high sensitivity (84–85.9%), specificity (99.8%), an acceptable ~3 operations per case of cancer detected and a 3% complication rate. ROCA doubled the number of OCs detected compared to a single absolute Ca125 threshold rule. Additionally ROCA-based multimodal screening was associated with a statistically significant stage shift of 14% towards early stage I/II/IIIa disease (40%) compared to controls (26%) ($P$ <0.0001) [76]. Although the primary Cox-proportional-hazards analysis did not show a significant mortality impact, secondary analyses using statistical adjustment for a potential delayed effect on mortality, found a statistically significant 23% (CI:1,46, $P$ = 0.021) delayed mortality benefit 7–14 years postrandomisation [76]. A delayed mortality benefit has also been reported in other (non-OC) screening trials. The UKCTOCS cohort is now being followed up for another 3 years to conclusively determine whether there is a delayed mortality benefit.

In high-risk women, 'annual' screening for OC using absolute CA125 and an ultrasound scan is not effective and not advocated. Phase-1 of UKFOCSS (United Kingdom Familial Ovarian Cancer Screening Study) reported an 81.3–87.5% sensitivity, 25.5% positive predictive value (PPV) and 99.9% negative predictive value (NPV) with annual screening [77]. A more frequent (3–4 monthly) longitudinal CA125-based ROCA-based screening strategy in high-risk women >35 years has subsequently been investigated in UKFOCSS Phase-2 (4,348 women; 13,728 women-screen-years) in the UK [78] and the Cancer Genetics Network (CGN) and Gynaecological Oncology Group (GOG) trials (3692 women, 13,080 women-screen-years) in the USA [79,80].

UKFOCSS-P2 results published recently show high sensitivity, PPV and NPV within one year of screening of 94.7%, 10.8%, and 100% respectively. Screening led to a significant stage shift. 7/19 (36.8%) of cancers diagnosed within 1 year of last screen were stage IIIb/IV compared with 17/18 (94.4%) cancers diagnosed >1 year after the last screen ($P$ = 0.001). Additionally, 95% of screen-detected cancers achieved a R0 resection (zero residual disease) at debulking surgery, an accepted surrogate for better survival. Similar findings were reported in the CGN/GOG studies. These data appear promising and suggest potential benefit of 4-monthly longitudinal CA125 algorithm based screening of high-risk women who decline risk-reducing surgery. A national screening programme for OC is unlikely to be considered before the UKCTOCS long-term follow-up data are reported. In the interim, in the UK, a new project evaluating 4-monthly ROCA-based screening in high-risk women, called ALDO (avoiding late diagnosis of ovarian cancer) has commenced in autumn of 2018. For OC-screening to be effective it is essential for gynaecologists/gynae-oncologists/multidisciplinary teams to change their approach by being willing to operate on the basis of a rising biomarker without radiological corroboration of any abnormality.

## Endometrial cancer screening

The evidence-base to EC-screening in high-risk women (LS/Cowden's syndrome) is limited and survival data are lacking. Nevertheless, screening could have a role to play in women who wish to delay surgical prevention, and is usually undertaken from 35 years. Inferences can be drawn from multiple cohort studies published in the literature [81–84]. EC-screening options involve annual transvaginal-ultrasound (TVS) and endometrial sampling alone or outpatient hysteroscopy plus endometrial sampling (OHES). TVS alone without endometrial sampling is not effective. Additionally women are advised to maintain a menstrual diary/calendar and any unscheduled or abnormal bleeding should be promptly investigated. Hysteroscopy-based screening has the advantage of endometrial visualisation and ability to take a targeted biopsy. Annual EC-screening can detect pre-invasive disease, i.e. atypical endometrial hyperplasia as well as early stage EC. Interval cancers have also been reported despite screening. Further well designed research studies evaluating the potential benefit of EC-screening in high-risk women are warranted.

# SURGICAL PREVENTION IN HIGH RISK WOMEN

## Risk reducing salpingo-oophorectomy

The gold-standard and most effective method of preventing OC in high-risk women once they have completed their family is RRSO. RRSO can reduce OC-risk by 80–96% in *BRCA1/BRCA2*-carriers, [85–88] but a 2–4% residual risk of primary-peritoneal cancer remains [89,90]. RRSO has been shown to reduce OC and all-cause mortality. Oophorectomy also reduces OC-risk by 94% in women at average/population-based risk of OC [91]. In *BRCA1*-carriers OC-risk begins to rise from 35 years age and increases significantly after the age of 40 years. In *BRCA2*-carriers, OC-risk rises from 40 years and increases significantly after 45 years. RRSO is usually offered from 35–40 years in *BRCA1* and 40–45 years in *BRCA2* carriers. It may be offered up to 5-year before the earliest onset of OC in the family. Although initial studies indicated a ~50% reduction in BC-risk from premenopausal oophorectomy [87,92,93], this has become contentious, as more recent data from Dutch study showed no benefit of reduction in BC-risk [94] and a Canadian study showed a reduction only in premenopausal *BRCA2* BC-risk [95]. Overall RRSO has high satisfaction rates (>85%) and leads to reduced cancer worry [96].

The standard RRSO procedure involves removal (usually laparoscopic) of both tubes and ovaries as well as peritoneal cytology/washings. It is essential that a serial sectioning 'SEE-FIM' protocol be used for pathological assessment [97]. Diathermy injury to the fimbrial end should be avoided [98]. Following RRSO around 5% women are found to have an occult in situ (STIC – serous tubular in situ carcinoma) lesion or microscopic invasive cancer at histological examination [99,100]. A number of these lesions would be missed without a 'SEE-FIM' protocol. Interestingly 70% of these occult lesions are tubal rather than ovarian [100]. Women found to have in situ/invasive cancer should be referred to the gynaeoncology MDT and may need a further full staging surgical procedure (see **Table 8.3** for current recommendations).

In premenopausal women, RRSO leads to premature surgical menopause. This is associated with an increased risk of osteoporosis, vasomotor symptoms, sexual dysfunction, cardiovascular disease, neurocognitive impairment and dementia [91,96,101,102]. These detrimental consequences can be ameliorated by hormone

### Table 8.3 Management of occult in situ or invasive cancer detected post RRSO

| Histopathology and cytology | Management |
| --- | --- |
| Invasive cancer +/− positive cytology* | • Staging CT<br>• Surgical staging |
| STIC with positive cytology* | • Staging CT<br>• Surgical staging. |
| STIC with negative cytology* | • Staging CT<br>• Surgical staging not indicated (unless abnormality on CT suggesting otherwise) |
| Normal histopathology with positive cytology* | • Staging CT<br>• Surgical staging |
| Normal histopathology with negative cytology | • No action required |

* Panel genetic-testing (BRCA1/BRCA2/RAD51C/ RAD51D/BRIP1) if not already undertaken

replacement therapy (HRT) and are mainly seen in those who undergo premature menopause <45 years and do not take HRT. Women who do not have a personal history of BC should be offered HRT until 51 years age (average age of menopause). Short-term HRT in this manner does not increase the BC-risk [103]. For women with a history of BC, HRT is usually contraindicated but this should be discussed with the breast oncology team.

The timing of RRSO needs to be individualised to the patient and decision-making can be a complex process [104]. Women should be adequately counselled on the pros and cons of RRSO, including the effects of iatrogenic menopause and its detrimental effects on cardiovascular, bone, neurological and psychosexual health [91,96,101,102]. There is a 3–5% complication rate reported in the literature [99]. The OC-risk threshold for RRSO was recently specified as >4% lifetime risk in premenopausal women and >5% lifetime risk in postmenopausal women as it is cost-effective above these levels of risk [105,106]. Hence, RRSO can also be offered to women at intermediate 5–10% risk of OC. This includes *RAD51C*, *RAD51D* and *BRIP1* mutation carriers as well as 'selected' women with a strong FH of 'BC and OC' or 'OC-alone' who have unknown mutation status or are *BRCA*-negative. Guidelines need revising to broaden access to RRSO so that a number of women who could not earlier access RRSO can benefit from surgical prevention [107]. In *RAD51C/RAD51D* carriers RRSO may be offered at >40 years and in *BRIP1* carriers at >50 years. Complex risk-models incorporating genetic (high/moderate penetrance genes and SNP/common genetic variants) data along with epidemiological information are being developed using sophisticated computational tools. These will provide women individualised OC-risk estimates. Once these are validated in the future they could provide a means to stratify a population by OC-risk and offer targeted surgical prevention.

## Early salpingectomy and delayed oophorectomy

With increasing evidence of the central role of the fallopian tube in the etiopathogenesis of epithelial-OC, initial bilateral-salpingectomy followed by delayed-oophorectomy has been proposed as an attractive two-stage surgical alternative to RRSO. This has the advantage of offering some level of risk-reduction to those women who decline or wish to delay RRSO whilst conserving ovarian function and avoiding detrimental consequences of early menopause [108-110]. However, prospective outcome data for risk-reducing early-salpingectomy and delayed-oophorectomy (RRESDO) are lacking. The precise level of risk-reduction and long-term consequences on ovarian function are unknown. Concerns have also been expressed regarding the potential attrition from delayed-oophorectomy. A proportion of women who do not undergo this may develop OC. Therefore, RRESDO in high-risk women should be currently offered only in the safe environment of a clinical trial and 80% of UK-clinicians are supportive of this [111]. Trials are currently underway in the Netherlands, France, USA and soon to commence in the UK.

## Lynch syndrome

Surgical prevention in LS women includes a total laparoscopic hysterectomy and bilateral salpingo-oophorectomy (TLH BSO), after completion of their family, usually after 40 years age [112]. Prophylactic TLH BSO has been reported to prevent EC and OC. The risk of primary peritoneal cancer postsurgery is very rare in this population (unlike *BRCA1/2*-carriers) with just couple of case-reports in the literature [113]. As highlighted earlier, HRT is recommended in premenopausal women till the age of 51 years.

## OTHER OPTIONS FOR RISK REDUCTION

Unaffected carriers can benefit from lifestyle advice which can reduce their risk of cancer such as contraceptive pill use, breastfeeding, planning a family, and PGD [114-116]. Five years use of the contraceptive pill can half the OC-risk in *BRCA1/BRCA2*-carriers [115]. The data on impact of pill use on BC-risk in *BRCA*-carriers are conflicting with some studies showing an increased risk and others no increase in risk. Pros and cons of contraceptive pill use need to be discussed with the patient and it can be given at earlier age when the absolute BC-risk is lower. It is contraindicated in women who have had BC. More intensive annual MRI screening for BC is advisable from 30 years and is available through specialist breast clinics [117]. BC chemoprevention options include Tamoxifen/Anastrazole [118,119]. Risk-reducing mastectomy can reduce BC-risk by >90% [62]. Aspirin is an effective option for chemoprevention for LS women. RCT data from the CAPP2 trial show aspirin reduces CRC and overall cancer risk in LS [65]. Colonoscopy every 1–2 years has shown a reduction in mortality from CRC by 63% [120].

> **Key points for Clinical Practice**
>
> - *BRCA1/BRCA2* mutations cause the majority of known inheritable OC risk. *BRCA1* carriers have a 44% and 71% risk of OC and BC respectively till 80 years of age. *BRCA2* carriers have a 17% and 69% risk of OC and BC respectively till 80 years.
> - *RAD51C, RAD51D* and *BRIP1* are recently validated moderate penetrance OC genes. OC risk with *RAD51C/RAD51D* is ~11% and *BRIP1* ~6%. They are not associated with an increased risk of BC.
> - The NICE recommends *BRCA1/BRCA2* testing be offered to individuals with a 10% combined *BRCA1/BRCA2* probability. Commonly used FH based risk models are MSS (not suitable for use in AJ families), BOADICEA, BRCAPRO, Tyrer-Cuzick.
> - Genetic-testing is now recommended for all high grade nonmucinous EOC and triple negative BC.

- FH-based prediction models are moderately effective at predicting *BRCA1/BRCA2* mutation and have a poor ability for predicting their absence. A population-based approach to testing which has been investigated in the AJ population has shown to identify 50% more people at risk, not adversely affect psychological health and is cost effective.
- IHC/MSI testing on tumour tissue for EC (and CRC) cases is recommended to increase ascertainment for LS. Genetic-testing is then recommended for those whose tumour tissue stains negative for MMR protein on IHC or tumour with an unstable MSI result.
- Advantages of genetic-testing include:
    - Use of targeted therapies (PARP inhibitors in *BRCA1/BRCA2* mutated platinum sensitive relapsed EOC).
    - Options of screening (MRI/mammography in women at increased BC-risk and hysteroscopy with endometrial biopsy and colonoscopies in LS).
    - Risk reducing surgery (RRSO/RRESDO for increased OC-risk; RRM for increased BC-risk and hysterectomy and BSO in LS).
    - Chemoprevention (SERMs for BC-risk, OCP for OC-risk and aspirin in LS).
    - Reproductive choices and PGD.
    - Predictive testing of family members.
- Disadvantages of genetic-testing include possible psychological distress, familial implications and potential implications for insurance/employability.
- Although at present OC screening in women at increased risk is not indicated outside the context of a clinical trial, data appear promising and suggest potential benefit of 4 monthly longitudinal CA125 algorithm based screening for women who decline risk reducing surgery.
- Although the evidence-base to EC screening in high risk women is limited and survival data lacking, it could have a role to play in women who wish to delay surgical prevention.
- Oophorectomy in premenopausal women results in premature menopause which has detrimental health sequelae such as an increased risk of CVD, osteoporosis, cognitive decline, vasomotor symptoms and impaired sexual function. HRT is recommended in individuals without a personal history of BC until the age of 51 years.
- RRSO is the current standard of care to prevent OC in individuals at increased risk.
- RRESDO is an alternative two staged surgical approach in women wishing to avoid the health consequences of premature menopause. This must only be offered in the context of a clinical trial as at present the precise level of risk reduction and long-term consequences on ovarian function are unknown.

## REFERENCES

1. Lichtenstein P, Holm NV, Verkasalo PK, et al. Environmental and heritable factors in the causation of cancer--analyses of cohorts of twins from Sweden, Denmark, and Finland. N Engl JMed 2000; 343:78–85.
2. George A, Riddell D, Seal S, et al. Implementing rapid, robust, cost-effective, patient-centred, routine genetic testing in ovarian cancer patients. Scientific reports 2016; 6:29506.
3. Song H, Cicek MS, Dicks E, et al. The contribution of deleterious germline mutations in BRCA1, BRCA2 and the mismatch repair genes to ovarian cancer in the population. Hum Mol Genet 2014; 23:4703–4709.
4. Jervis S, Song H, Lee A, et al. A risk prediction algorithm for ovarian cancer incorporating BRCA1, BRCA2, common alleles and other familial effects. J Med Gen 2015; 52:465–475.
5. Jervis S, Song H, Lee A, et al. Ovarian cancer familial relative risks by tumour subtypes and by known ovarian cancer genetic susceptibility variants. J Med Genet 2014; 51:108–113.
6. Hampel H, Frankel W, Panescu J, et al. Screening for Lynch syndrome (hereditary nonpolyposis colorectal cancer) among endometrial cancer patients. Cancer research 2006; 66:7810–7817.

# References

7. Batte BA, Bruegl AS, Daniels MS, et al. Consequences of universal MSI/IHC in screening ENDOMETRIAL cancer patients for Lynch syndrome. Gynecol Oncol 2014; 134:319–325.
8. Ferguson SE, Aronson M, Pollett A, et al. Performance characteristics of screening strategies for Lynch syndrome in unselected women with newly diagnosed endometrial cancer who have undergone universal germline mutation testing. Cancer 2014; 120:3932–3939.
9. Moline J, Mahdi H, Yang B, et al. Implementation of tumor testing for lynch syndrome in endometrial cancers at a large academic medical center. Gynecol Oncol 2013; 130:121–126.
10. Minion LE, Dolinsky JS, Chase DM, et al. Hereditary predisposition to ovarian cancer, looking beyond BRCA1/BRCA2. Gynecol Oncol 2015; 137:86–92.
11. Pal T, Akbari MR, Sun P, et al. Frequency of mutations in mismatch repair genes in a population-based study of women with ovarian cancer. Br J Cancer 2012; 107:1783–1790.
12. Meyer LA, Broaddus RR, Lu KH. Endometrial cancer and Lynch syndrome: clinical and pathologic considerations. Cancer Control 2009; 16:14–22.
13. Ring KL, Garcia C, Thomas MH, et al. Current and future role of genetic screening in gynecologic malignancies. American journal of obstetrics and gynecology 2017; 217:512–521. 14. Barrow E, Hill J, Evans DG. Cancer risk in Lynch syndrome. Familial Cancer 2013; 12:229–240.
15. Manchanda R, Loggenberg K, Sanderson S, et al. Population testing for cancer predisposing BRCA1/BRCA2 mutations in the Ashkenazi-Jewish community: a randomized controlled trial. J Natli Cancer Inst 2015; 107:379.
16. Ferla R, Calo V, Cascio S, et al. Founder mutations in BRCA1 and BRCA2 genes. Ann Oncol 2007; 18:vi93–98.
17. Kuchenbaecker KB, Hopper JL, Barnes DR, et al. Risks of Breast, Ovarian, and Contralateral Breast Cancer for BRCA1 and BRCA2 Mutation Carriers. JAMA 2017; 317:2402–2416. 18. Liede A, Karlan BY, Narod SA. Cancer risks for male carriers of germline mutations in BRCA1 or BRCA2: a review of the literature. J Clin Oncol 2004; 22:735–742.
19. Roed Nielsen H, Petersen J, Therkildsen C, et al. Increased risk of male cancer and identification of a potential prostate cancer cluster region in BRCA2. Acta Oncol 2016; 55:38–44.
20. Petersen GM. Familial pancreatic cancer. Semin Oncol 2016; 43:548–553.
21. Loveday C, Turnbull C, Ramsay E, et al. Germline mutations in RAD51D confer susceptibility to ovarian cancer. Nat Genet 2011; 43:879–882.
22. Loveday C, Turnbull C, Ruark E, et al. Germline RAD51C mutations confer susceptibility to ovarian cancer. Nat Genet 2012; 44:475–476.
23. Ramus SJ, Song H, Dicks E, et al. Germline Mutations in the BRIP1, BARD1, PALB2, and NBN Genes in Women With Ovarian Cancer. J Natl Cancer Inst 2015; 107.
24. Vasen HF, Moslein G, Alonso A, et al. Guidelines for the clinical management of Lynch syndrome (hereditary non-polyposis cancer). J Med Genet 2007; 44:353–362.
25. Bubien V, Bonnet F, Brouste V, et al. High cumulative risks of cancer in patients with PTEN hamartoma tumour syndrome. J Med Genet 2013; 50:255–263.
26. Tan MH, Mester JL, Ngeow J, et al. Lifetime cancer risks in individuals with germline PTEN mutations. Clin Cancer Res 2012; 18:400–407. 27. Hearle N, Schumacher V, Menko FH, et al. Frequency and spectrum of cancers in the Peutz-Jeghers syndrome. Clin Cancer Res 2006; 12:3209–3215.
28. Beggs AD, Latchford AR, Vasen HF, et al. Peutz-Jeghers syndrome: a systematic review and recommendations for management. Gut 2010; 59:975–986. 29. Evans DG, Harkness EF, Plaskocinska I, et al. Pathology update to the Manchester Scoring System based on testing in over 4000 families. J Med Genet 2017; 54:674–681.
30. Bredart A, Kop JL, Antoniou AC, et al. Use of the BOADICEA Web Application in clinical practice: appraisals by clinicians from various countries. Fam Cancer 2017.
31. Mazzola E, Blackford A, Parmigiani G, et al. Recent Enhancements to the Genetic Risk Prediction Model BRCAPRO. Cancer informatics 2015; 14:147–157.
32. National Collaborating Centre for C. National Institute for Health and Clinical Excellence: Guidance. Familial Breast Cancer: Classification and Care of People at Risk of Familial Breast Cancer and Management of Breast Cancer and Related Risks in People with a Family History of Breast Cancer. Cardiff (UK): National Collaborating Centre for Cancer (UK). National Collaborating Centre for Cancer, 2013.
33. Kang HH, Williams R, Leary J, et al. Evaluation of models to predict BRCA germline mutations. British journal of cancer 2006; 95:914–920.
34. Gabai-Kapara E, Lahad A, Kaufman B, et al. Population-based screening for breast and ovarian cancer risk due to BRCA1 and BRCA2. Proceedings of the National Academy of Sciences of the United States of America 2014; 111:14205–14210. 35. King MC, Marks JH, Mandell JB. Breast and ovarian cancer risks due to inherited mutations in BRCA1 and BRCA2. Science (New York, NY) 2003; 302:643–646.

36. Moller P, Hagen AI, Apold J, et al. Genetic epidemiology of BRCA mutations – family history detects less than 50% of the mutation carriers. European journal of cancer (Oxford, England : 1990) 2007; 43:1713–1717.
37. ACOG Practice Bulletin No. 147: Lynch syndrome. Obstetrics and gynecology 2014; 124:1042–1054.
38. Hampel H, Frankel WL, Martin E, et al. Screening for the Lynch syndrome (hereditary nonpolyposis colorectal cancer). N Engl J Med 2005; 352:1851–1860.
39. Umar A, Boland CR, Terdiman JP, et al. Revised Bethesda Guidelines for hereditary nonpolyposis colorectal cancer (Lynch syndrome) and microsatellite instability. J Natl Cancer Inst 2004; 96:261–268.
40. Pinol V, Castells A, Andreu M, et al. Accuracy of revised Bethesda guidelines, microsatellite instability, and immunohistochemistry for the identification of patients with hereditary nonpolyposis colorectal cancer. JAMA 2005; 293:1986–1994.
41. Vasen HF, Blanco I, Aktan-Collan K, et al. Revised guidelines for the clinical management of Lynch syndrome (HNPCC): recommendations by a group of European experts. Gut 2013; 62:812–823.
42. Kwon JS, Scott JL, Gilks CB, et al. Testing women with endometrial cancer to detect Lynch syndrome. J Clin Oncol 2011; 29:2247–2252. 43. Mvundura M, Grosse SD, Hampel H, et al. The cost-effectiveness of genetic testing strategies for Lynch syndrome among newly diagnosed patients with colorectal cancer. Genet Med 2010; 12:93–104.
44. Nelson HD, Pappas M, Zakher B, et al. Risk assessment, genetic counseling, and genetic testing for BRCA-related cancer in women: a systematic review to update the U.S. Preventive Services Task Force recommendation. Ann Int Med 2014; 160:255–266.
45. Robson ME, Bradbury AR, Arun B, et al. American Society of Clinical Oncology Policy Statement Update: Genetic and Genomic Testing for Cancer Susceptibility. J Clin Oncol 2015; 33:3660–3667.
46. Lancaster JM, Powell CB, Chen LM, et al. Society of Gynecologic Oncology statement on risk assessment for inherited gynecologic cancer predispositions. Gynecol Oncol 2015; 136:3–7.
47. Walsh T, Casadei S, Lee MK, et al. Mutations in 12 genes for inherited ovarian, fallopian tube, and peritoneal carcinoma identified by massively parallel sequencing. Proceedings of the National Academy of Sciences of the United States of America 2011; 108:18032–18037.
48. Buys SS, Sandbach JF, Gammon A, et al. A study of over 35,000 women with breast cancer tested with a 25-gene panel of hereditary cancer genes. Cancer 2017; 123:1721–1730.
49. Couch FJ, Hart SN, Sharma P, et al. Inherited mutations in 17 breast cancer susceptibility genes among a large triple-negative breast cancer cohort unselected for family history of breast cancer. Journal of clinical oncology : official journal of the American Society of Clinical Oncology 2015; 33:304–311.
50. NHS England. Clinical Commissioning Policy: Genetic Testing for BRCA1 and BRCA2 Mutations. 2015 03/2015. https://www.engage.england.nhs.uk/consultation/specialised-services-consultation/user_uploads/brca-policy.pdf (accessed 01/05/2015).
51. Kinney AY, Butler KM, Schwartz MD, et al. Expanding access to BRCA1/2 genetic counseling with telephone delivery: a cluster randomized trial. J Natl Cancer Inst 2014; 106.
52. Manchanda R, Burnell M, Loggenberg K, et al. Cluster-randomised non-inferiority trial comparing DVD-assisted and traditional genetic counselling in systematic population testing for BRCA1/2 mutations. J Med Genet 2016; 53:472–480.
53. Schwartz MD, Valdimarsdottir HB, Peshkin BN, et al. Randomized noninferiority trial of telephone versus in-person genetic counseling for hereditary breast and ovarian cancer. J Clin Oncol 2014; 32:618–626.
54. Systematic genetic testing for personalised ovarian cancer therapy (SIGNPOST). 2017. https://www.isrctn.com/ISRCTN16988857?q=&filters=conditionCategory:Cancer&sort=&offset=4&totalResults=1950&page=1&pageSize=10&searchType=basic-search (accessed 8.10.2017).
55. Ledermann J, Harter P, Gourley C, et al. Olaparib maintenance therapy in patients with platinum-sensitive relapsed serous ovarian cancer: a preplanned retrospective analysis of outcomes by BRCA status in a randomised phase 2 trial. Lancet Oncol 2014; 15:852–861.
56. Ledermann JA, Harter P, Gourley C, et al. Overall survival in patients with platinum-sensitive recurrent serous ovarian cancer receiving olaparib maintenance monotherapy: an updated analysis from a randomised, placebo-controlled, double-blind, phase 2 trial. Lancet Oncol 2016; 17:1579–1589.
57. EMA. EPAR summary for the public. Lynparza (olaparib) 2015. http://www.ema.europa.eu/docs/en_GB/document_library/EPAR_-_Summary_for_the_public/human/003726/WC500180153.pdf.
58. FDA. FDA approves Lynparza to treat advanced ovarian cancer, 2014.
59. NICE. Olaparib for maintenance treatment of relapsed, platinum-sensitive, BRCA mutation-positive ovarian, fallopian tube and peritoneal cancer after response to second-line or subsequent platinum-based chemotherap. National Institute for Health and Care Excellence, London, UK 2016.

60. Finch A, Beiner M, Lubinski J, et al. Salpingo-oophorectomy and the risk of ovarian, fallopian tube, and peritoneal cancers in women with a BRCA1 or BRCA2 Mutation. JAMA 2006; 296:185–192.
61. Rebbeck TR, Kauff ND, Domchek SM. Meta-analysis of risk reduction estimates associated with risk-reducing salpingo-oophorectomy in BRCA1 or BRCA2 mutation carriers. J Natl Cancer Inst 2009; 101:80–87.
62. Rebbeck TR, Friebel T, Lynch HT, et al. Bilateral prophylactic mastectomy reduces breast cancer risk in BRCA1 and BRCA2 mutation carriers: the PROSE Study Group. J Clin Oncol 2004; 22:1055–1062.
63. Cuzick J, Sestak I, Bonanni B, et al. Selective oestrogen receptor modulators in prevention of breast cancer: an updated meta-analysis of individual participant data. Lancet 2013; 381:1827–1834.
64. Menon U, Harper J, Sharma A, et al. Views of BRCA gene mutation carriers on preimplantation genetic diagnosis as a reproductive option for hereditary breast and ovarian cancer. Hum Reprod 2007.
65. Burn J, Gerdes AM, Macrae F, et al. Long-term effect of aspirin on cancer risk in carriers of hereditary colorectal cancer: an analysis from the CAPP2 randomised controlled trial. Lancet 2011; 378:2081–2087.
66. Rothwell PM, Fowkes FG, Belch JF, et al. Effect of daily aspirin on long-term risk of death due to cancer: analysis of individual patient data from randomised trials. Lancet 2011; 377:31–41.
67. Rothwell PM, Price JF, Fowkes FG, et al. Short-term effects of daily aspirin on cancer incidence, mortality, and non-vascular death: analysis of the time course of risks and benefits in 51 randomised controlled trials. Lancet 2012; 379:1602–1612.
68. Metcalfe KA, Poll A, Royer R, et al. Screening for founder mutations in BRCA1 and BRCA2 in unselected Jewish women. J Clin Oncol 2010; 28:387–391.
69. Manchanda R, Legood R, Burnell M, et al. Cost-effectiveness of population screening for BRCA mutations in Ashkenazi jewish women compared with family history-based testing. J Natl Cancer Inst 2015; 107:380.
70. Manchanda R, Jacobs I. Genetic screening for gynecological cancer: where are we heading? Future Oncol 2015.
71. PROMISE - Predicting Risk of Ovarian Malignancy, Improved Screening and Early detection. 2016. https://eveappeal.org.uk/our-research/our-research-programmes/promise-2016/ (accessed 03/08/2016).
72. Jacobs IJ, Skates SJ, MacDonald N, et al. Screening for ovarian cancer: a pilot randomised controlled trial. Lancet 1999; 353:1207–1210.
73. Kobayashi H, Yamada Y, Sado T, et al. A randomized study of screening for ovarian cancer: a multicenter study in Japan. International J Gynecol Cancer2008;18:414–420.
74. Buys SS, Partridge E, Black A, et al. Effect of screening on ovarian cancer mortality: the Prostate, Lung, Colorectal and Ovarian (PLCO) Cancer Screening Randomized Controlled Trial. JAMA 2011; 305:2295–2303.
75. Buys SS, Partridge E, Black A, et al. Effect of screening on ovarian cancer mortality: the Prostate, Lung, Colorectal and Ovarian (PLCO) Cancer Screening Randomized Controlled Trial. JAMA 2011; 305:2295–2303.
76. Jacobs IJ, Menon U, Ryan A, et al. Ovarian cancer screening and mortality in the UK Collaborative Trial of Ovarian Cancer Screening (UKCTOCS): a randomised controlled trial. Lancet 2016; 387:945–956. 77. Rosenthal AN, Fraser L, Manchanda R, et al. Results of annual screening in phase I of the United Kingdom familial ovarian cancer screening study highlight the need for strict adherence to screening schedule. J Clin Oncol 2013; 31:49–57.
78. Rosenthal AN, Fraser LSM, Philpott S, et al. Evidence of Stage Shift in Women Diagnosed With Ovarian Cancer During Phase II of the United Kingdom Familial Ovarian Cancer Screening Study. J Clin Oncol 2017; 35:1411–1420. 79. Greene MH, Piedmonte M, Alberts D, et al. A prospective study of risk-reducing salpingo-oophorectomy and longitudinal CA-125 screening among women at increased genetic risk of ovarian cancer: design and baseline characteristics: a gynecologic oncology group study. Cancer Epidemiol Biomarkers Prev 2008; 17:594–604.
80. Skates SJ, Greene MH, Buys SS, et al. Early Detection of Ovarian Cancer using the Risk of Ovarian Cancer Algorithm with Frequent CA125 Testing in Women at Increased Familial Risk - Combined Results from Two Screening Trials. Clin Cancer Res 2017.81. Dove-Edwin I, Boks D, Goff S, et al. The outcome of endometrial carcinoma surveillance by ultrasound scan in women at risk of hereditary nonpolyposis colorectal carcinoma and familial colorectal carcinoma. Cancer 2002; 94:1708–1712. 82. Gerritzen LH, Hoogerbrugge N, Oei AL, et al. Improvement of endometrial biopsy over transvaginal ultrasound alone for endometrial surveillance in women with Lynch syndrome. Fam Cancer 2009; 8:391–397. 83. Manchanda R, Saridogan E, Abdelraheim A, et al. Annual outpatient hysteroscopy and endometrial sampling (OHES) in HNPCC/Lynch syndrome (LS). Archives of gynecology and obstetrics 2012; 286:1555–1562.

84. Renkonen-Sinisalo L, Butzow R, Leminen A, et al. Surveillance for endometrial cancer in hereditary nonpolyposis colorectal cancer syndrome. Int J Cancer 2007; 120:821–824.
85. Kauff ND, Satagopan JM, Robson ME, et al. Risk-reducing salpingo-oophorectomy in women with a BRCA1 or BRCA2 mutation. N Engl J Med 2002; 346:1609–1615.
86. Rebbeck TR, Lynch HT, Neuhausen SL, et al. Prophylactic oophorectomy in carriers of BRCA1 or BRCA2 mutations. N Engl J Med 2002; 346:1616–1622. 8
87. Kauff ND, Domchek SM, Friebel TM, et al. Risk-reducing salpingo-oophorectomy for the prevention of BRCA1- and BRCA2-associated breast and gynecologic cancer: a multicenter, prospective study. J Clin Oncol 2008; 26:1331–1337.
88. Finch A, Beiner M, Lubinski J, et al. Salpingo-oophorectomy and the risk of ovarian, fallopian tube, and peritoneal cancers in women with a BRCA1 or BRCA2 Mutation. JAMA 2006; 296:185–192.
89. Finch A, Shaw P, Rosen B, et al. Clinical and pathologic findings of prophylactic salpingo-oophorectomies in 159 BRCA1 and BRCA2 carriers. Gynecol Oncol 2006;100:58–64.
90. Casey MJ, Synder C, Bewtra C, et al. Intra-abdominal carcinomatosis after prophylactic oophorectomy in women of hereditary breast ovarian cancer syndrome kindreds associated with BRCA1 and BRCA2 mutations. Gynecol Oncol 2005; 97:457–467.
91. Parker WH, Feskanich D, Broder MS, et al. Long-term mortality associated with oophorectomy compared with ovarian conservation in the nurses' health study. Obstet Gynecol 2013; 121:709–716. 92. Domchek SM, Friebel TM, Singer CF, et al. Association of risk-reducing surgery in BRCA1 or BRCA2 mutation carriers with cancer risk and mortality. JAMA 2010; 304:967–975.
93. Chai X, Domchek S, Kauff N, et al. RE: Breast Cancer Risk After Salpingo-Oophorectomy in Healthy BRCA1/2 Mutation Carriers: Revisiting the Evidence for Risk Reduction. J Natl Cancer Inst 2015; 107.
94. Heemskerk-Gerritsen BA, Seynaeve C, van Asperen CJ, et al. Breast cancer risk after salpingo-oophorectomy in healthy BRCA1/2 mutation carriers: revisiting the evidence for risk reduction. J Natl Cancer Inst 2015; 107.
95. Kotsopoulos J, Huzarski T, Gronwald J, et al. Bilateral Oophorectomy and Breast Cancer Risk in BRCA1 and BRCA2 Mutation Carriers. J Natl Cancer Inst 2017; 109.
96. Madalinska JB, Hollenstein J, Bleiker E, et al. Quality-of-life effects of prophylactic salpingo-oophorectomy versus gynecologic screening among women at increased risk of hereditary ovarian cancer. J Clin Oncol 2005; 23:6890–6898.
97. Medeiros F, Muto MG, Lee Y, et al. The tubal fimbria is a preferred site for early adenocarcinoma in women with familial ovarian cancer syndrome. Am J Surg Pathol 2006; 30:230–6.
98. Manchanda R, Silvanto A, Abdelraheim A, et al. Diathermy-induced injury may affect detection of occult tubal lesions at risk-reducing salpingo-oophorectomy. Int J Gynecol Cancer 2012; 22:881–888. 99. Manchanda R, Abdelraheim A, Johnson M, et al. Outcome of risk-reducing salpingo-oophorectomy in BRCA carriers and women of unknown mutation status. BJOG 2011; 118:814–824.
100. Powell CB. Risk reducing salpingo-oophorectomy for BRCA mutation carriers: twenty years later. Gynecol Oncol 2014; 132:261–263.
101. Madalinska JB, van Beurden M, Bleiker EM, et al. The impact of hormone replacement therapy on menopausal symptoms in younger high-risk women after prophylactic salpingo-oophorectomy. J Clin Oncol 2006; 24:3576–3582.
102. Rocca WA, Bower JH, Maraganore DM, et al. Increased risk of cognitive impairment or dementia in women who underwent oophorectomy before menopause. Neurology 2007; 69(:1074–1083.
103. Kotsopoulos J, Huzarski T, Gronwald J, et al. Hormone replacement therapy after menopause and risk of breast cancer in BRCA1 mutation carriers: a case-control study. Breast Cancer Res Treat 2016; 155:365–373. 104. Manchanda R, Burnell M, Abdelraheim A, et al. Factors influencing uptake and timing of risk reducing salpingo-oophorectomy in women at risk of familial ovarian cancer: a competing risk time to event analysis. BJOG 2012. 105. Manchanda R, Legood R, Antoniou AC, et al. Specifying the ovarian cancer risk threshold of 'premenopausal risk-reducing salpingo-oophorectomy' for ovarian cancer prevention: a cost-effectiveness analysis. Journal of medical genetics 2016; 53:591–599.
106. Manchanda R, Legood R, Pearce L, et al. Defining the risk threshold for risk reducing salpingo-oophorectomy for ovarian cancer prevention in low risk postmenopausal women. Gynecologic oncology 2015; 139:487–494.
107. Manchanda R, Legood R, Antoniou AC, et al. Commentary on changing the risk threshold for surgical prevention of ovarian cancer. BJOG 2017
108. Schenberg T, Mitchell G. Prophylactic bilateral salpingectomy as a prevention strategy in women at high-risk of ovarian cancer: a mini-review. Front Oncol 2014; 4:21.

109. McAlpine JN, Hanley GE, Woo MM, et al. Opportunistic salpingectomy: uptake, risks, and complications of a regional initiative for ovarian cancer prevention. Am J Obstet Gynecol 2014; 210:471.e1–11.
110. Kwon JS, McAlpine JN, Hanley GE, et al. Costs and benefits of opportunistic salpingectomy as an ovarian cancer prevention strategy. Obstet Gynecol 2015; 125:338–345.
111. Chandrasekaran D, Menon U, Evans G, et al. Risk reducing salpingectomy and delayed oophorectomy in high risk women: views of cancer geneticists, genetic counsellors and gynaecological oncologists in the UK. Fam Cancer 2015; 14:521–530.
112. Schmeler KM, Lynch HT, Chen LM, et al. Prophylactic surgery to reduce the risk of gynecologic cancers in the Lynch syndrome. N Engl J Med 2006; 354:261–269.
113. Ghezzi F, Uccella S, Cromi A, et al. Primary peritoneal cancer in Lynch syndrome: a clinical-pathologic report of a case and analysis of the literature. Int J Gynecol Pathol 2013; 32:163–166.
114. Menon U, Harper J, Sharma A, et al. Views of BRCA gene mutation carriers on preimplantation genetic diagnosis as a reproductive option for hereditary breast and ovarian cancer. Hum Reprod 2007; 22:1573–1577.
115. Friebel TM, Domchek SM, Rebbeck TR. Modifiers of cancer risk in BRCA1 and BRCA2 mutation carriers: systematic review and meta-analysis. Journal of the National Cancer Institute 2014; 106:dju091.
116. Derks-Smeets IA, de Die-Smulders CE, Mackens S, et al. Hereditary breast and ovarian cancer and reproduction: an observational study on the suitability of preimplantation genetic diagnosis for both asymptomatic carriers and breast cancer survivors. Breast Cancer Res Treat 2014; 145:673–681.
117. NICE. Familial Breast Cancer: Classification and care of people at of familial breast cancer and management of breast cancer and related risks in people with a family history of breast cancer. National Institute for Health and Care Excellence, London, UK 2013(CG164).
118. Cuzick J, Sestak I, Forbes JF, et al. Anastrozole for prevention of breast cancer in high-risk postmenopausal women (IBIS-II): an international, double-blind, randomised placebo-controlled trial. Lancet 2014; 383:1041–1048.
119. Cuzick J, Forbes JF, Sestak I, et al. Long-term results of tamoxifen prophylaxis for breast cancer–96-month follow-up of the randomized IBIS-I trial. J Natl Cancer Inst 2007; 99:272–282.
120. Jarvinen HJ, Aarnio M, Mustonen H, et al. Controlled 15-year trial on screening for colorectal cancer in families with hereditary nonpolyposis colorectal cancer. Gastroenterology 2000; 118:829–834.
121. Evans DG, Lalloo F, Wallace A, Rahman N. Update on the Manchester Scoring System for BRCA1 and BRCA2 testing. J Med Genet 2005; 42:e39.
122. Network UGT. UK Genetic Testing Network Referral Criteria [Available from: https://ukgtn.nhs.uk/fileadmin/uploads/ukgtn/Documents/Resources/Library/Reports_Guidelines/UKGTN%20breast%20cancer%20Final%20161014.pdf
123 Genetics GC. GOSH Clinical Genetics Referral Guidelines [Available from: http://www.gosh.nhs.uk/health-professionals/clinical-specialties/clinical-genetics-information-health-professionals/refer-patient-genetics-department
124 Gan M, Manchanda. Screening in gynaecological cancers. In: (Ed) GM, ed. Textbook of Gynaecological Oncology 2016.
125. Evans DG, Harkness EF, Plaskocinska I, et al. Pathology update to the Manchester Scoring System based on testing in over 4000 families. J Med Genet 2017; 54:674–681.
126. Manchanda R, Abdelraheim A, Johnson M, et al. Outcome of risk-reducing salpingo-oophorectomy in BRCA carriers and women of unknown mutation status. BJOG 2011; 118:814–824.

# Chapter 9

# Vulval cancer in elderly women

*Madeleine Macdonald, John Tidy*

## INTRODUCTION

Although vulval cancer is uncommon, accounting for <1% of all cancer diagnoses in women each year, the incidence is rising; having increased in the UK by 10% over the last few decades [1,2]. In the US almost 6000 women were diagnosed with vulval cancer in 2016 [3]. The majority of women with vulval cancer are aged 70 years or over with the highest rates in those over 90 years old (see **Figure 9.1** with permission from Cancer Research UK).

Over 90% of vulval cancers are squamous cell carcinomas [4]. Unlike in younger women where high-risk human papilloma virus is the most common causal factor, in older women lichen sclerosus (LS) is the most frequent precursor. Approximately 4% of women with LS develop carcinoma with preinvasive differentiated vulval intraepithelial neoplasia (d-VIN) preceding the invasive disease [4]. Very rare forms of vulval cancer include vulval melanoma, basal cell cancer, Bartholin gland cancers and cancers of the apocrine glands. **Table 9.1** gives details of the staging of vulval cancer [5].

## STANDARD MANAGEMENT OF VULVAL CANCER

Management depends on stage of the disease, patient factors such as significant co-morbidities and patient wishes. For the earliest stage of disease (1a), a wide local excision with adequate disease-free margins is all that is required. The risk of recurrence is dependent on the disease-free margins; if >8 mm risk of recurrence is 0%, if <8 mm recurrence risk is up to 47% [4]. For stage 1b tumours as well as undertaking a wide radical excision (aiming for a surgical disease-free margin of 15 mm) dissection of the inguinal nodes (usually bilateral) is performed through separate groin incisions; a triple incision vulvectomy. Indication for lymphadenectomy is based on depth of invasion and maximum diameter of the tumour. If tumour depth is <1 mm and maximum diameter is 2 cm or less risk of lymph node metastases is negligible, however, in women with stage 1b disease risk of inguinal lymph node metastases is between 25–35% [6]. In patients with a lateral tumour 4 cm or more from the midline unilateral groin node dissection can be performed [4].

---

**Madeleine Macdonald** MRCOG, Subspecialty Trainee in Gynaecological Oncology, Jessop Wing, Royal Hallamshire Hospital, Sheffield, South Yorkshire, UK.

**John Tidy** MSc MD MBBS (Medicine), Professor and Consultant in Gynaecological Oncology, Royal Hallamshire Hospital, Sheffield, South Yorkshire, UK.

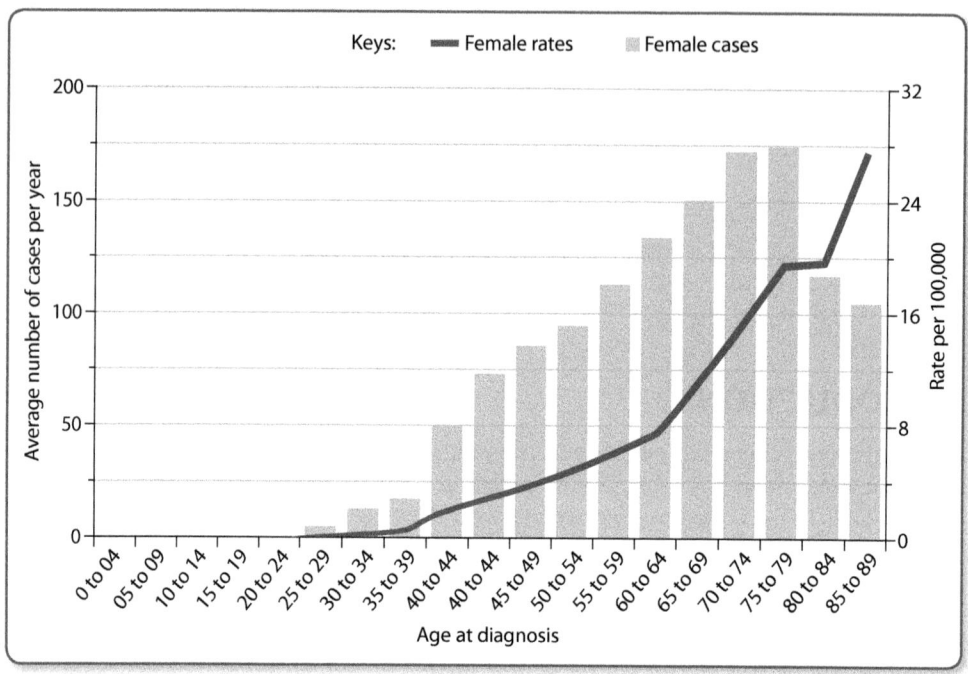

**Figure 9.1** Average number of new cases each year and age-specific incidence rates per 100,000 population, females, UK, reproduced with permission from Cancer Research UK [1].

| Table 9.1 Staging of vulval cancer [6] | |
|---|---|
| Stage | Description |
| Stage 1 | Tumour confined to the vulva |
| • 1a | • Lesions ≤2 cm in size, confined to the vulva or perineum and with stromal invasion ≤1 mm. No nodal metastasis |
| • 1b | • Lesions >2 cm in size or with stromal invasion >1 mm confined to the vulva or perineum. No nodal metastasis |
| Stage 2 | Tumour of any size with extension to adjacent perineal structures (lower 1/3 urethra; lower 1/3 vagina; anus) with negative nodes |
| Stage 3 | Tumour of any size with or without extension to adjacent perineal structures (lower 1/3 urethra; lower 1/3 vagina; anus) with positive inguinofemoral nodes |
| • IIIa | i. With 1 lymph node metastasis (≥5 mm), or<br>ii. 1–2 lymph node metastasis(es) (<5 mm) |
| • IIIb | i. With 2 or more lymph node metastases (≥5 mm), or<br>ii. 3 or more lymph node metastases (<5 mm) |
| • IIIc | With positive nodes with extracapsular spread |
| Stage 4 | Tumour invades other regional (upper 2/3 urethra; 2/3 vagina) or distant structures |
| • IVa | Tumour invades any of the following:<br>i. Upper urethral and/or vaginal mucosa; bladder mucosa; rectal mucosa or fixed to pelvic bone, or<br>ii. Fixed or ulcerated inguinofemoral lymph nodes |
| • IVb | Any distant metastasis including pelvic lymph nodes |

Morbidity related to surgery depends on the radicality of the procedure performed but includes wound problems; breakdown (20–40% of patients) [6] or infection, urinary or faecal incontinence, vulval scarring causing dyspareunia and psychosexual problems [4], and particular to groin node dissection lymphocysts and lymphoedema, reported to occur in 30–70% of patients [6]. Strategies to reduce the risk of groin wound problems and lower limb lymphoedema include preserving the saphenous vein and sentinel lymph node (SLN) biopsy, a procedure performed for many years for breast cancer [4]. The value of SLN biopsy rather than full lymphadenectomy for early stage vulval cancer continues to be investigated by the major international trial, The GROningen INternational Study on Sentinel nodes in Vulvar cancer (GROINSS-V) [6]. The original study published in 2008 reported, for tumours <4 cm in diameter and >1 mm deep, a 97% disease specific survival rate at 3 years for women with negative SLN concluding it was safe and feasible to omit full inguinal lymphadenectomy if the SLN was negative [6]. Morbidity, including wound breakdown, cellulitis and length of hospital stay, in the women who underwent SLN biopsy only was significantly reduced. Ten years follow-up results recently published by the group confirmed the safety of this approach with a 91% 10-year disease specific survival for patients with a negative SLN versus 65% for those with a positive SLN [7]. Isolated groin recurrence at 5 years was 2.5% for those with a negative SLN compared to 8% for those with a positive SLN. Similar results have been reported by Levenback et al in the GOG-173 study [8]. For women with positive sentinel nodes the ongoing GROINS-V II aims to assess if radiotherapy with or without chemotherapy is a safe alternative to full inguinal lymphadenectomy [9].

In patients with multiple co-morbidities who have significant symptoms especially severe vulval discomfort, a palliative excision of the vulval tumour only in order to improve their quality of life (QoL) may be an appropriate strategy.

For more advanced disease or recurrence in the vulva surgical management may involve a multidisciplinary team including plastic surgeons for reconstructive surgery using skin grafting or myocutaneous flaps and colorectal surgeons if part of the anus or anal sphincter is involved in the dissection in which cases a defunctioning colostomy may be necessary. A suprapubic catheter may be required if the urethra is involved or formation of an ileal conduit if a cystectomy is required.

Alternative management for recurrence or advanced disease is radiotherapy, with or without chemotherapy. In some instances radiotherapy may also be used for early stage tumours in close proximity to the anal sphincter as a primary treatment to preserve bowel function [4]. Morbidity from radical radiotherapy includes cystitis, proctitis, skin soreness, erythema and breakdown as well as generally fatigue.

## SURVIVAL AFTER VULVAL CANCER

Overall survival for vulval cancer has been improving steadily in the UK since 1970s with a 38% reduction in mortality rate over this time period, although over the last decade the rate has remained stable at 64% 5-year survival [1]. In the US, however, death rates from vulval cancer have increased slightly in recent years [3]. Overall 5-year survival rates for each stage reported by the International Federation of Gynaecology and Obstetrics (FIGO) can be seen in **Table 9.2**.

| Table 9.2 Five-year survival for each stage of vulval cancer [8] ||
|---|---|
| Stage | Five-year survival |
| Stage 1 | 80% |
| Stage 2 | 60% |
| Stage 3 | 40% |
| Stage 4 | 15% |

## CANCER AND THE ELDERLY

In 'medical terms' the age at which a patient becomes 'elderly' is currently 65 years of age. Further categorisation of elderly patients is often used for example 'younger-old' (65–74 years), 'older-old' (75–84 years) and 'oldest-old' (85 years and above) [10]. These subcategories can be useful in helping to predict morbidities and outcomes for patients. Evidence suggests the body's physiology alters significantly over 75 years old especially with regards to renal and hepatic function, body fat composition (increases) and water content (decreases), all of which may impact on a patient's ability to recovery from surgery or tolerance of radiotherapy or chemotherapy [10]. Many studies detail how the biological behaviour of disease including cancer differs in patients over 75 years and how patient's perception of the disease, and treatments available may influence management [10]; however, concerns have also been raised regarding clinicians attitudes towards treating older people with cancer and how this may have a significant negative impact on cancer survival in this group of patients [11].

Worldwide the percentage of people aged 65 years and older is increasing; in Japan it is estimated between 2000 and 2050 the numbers of young and working-age people will decline by 40%. Less dramatic declines are also predicted in China and Europe [12]. In the UK, census data reports the numbers of very elderly people (aged 85 years or more) increased by around 25% from 2001 to 2011 and two-thirds of this population are women [13]. Prompted by these changes in the population governments and international agencies such as the World Health Organisation (WHO), have begun to focus on the treatment of elderly patients with cancer [11,14]. As aforementioned concerns regarding equity in the access to curative treatments and healthcare professionals' attitudes towards treating older patients have been raised. Evidence suggests in all patients with cancer aged 75 years and over, rates of investigations and standard treatments fall [11]. Cancer Research UK found the rate of standard management for stage 1 vulval tumours declines with age; in women aged 65–74 years old and 75–84 years old; 75% and 73% respectively underwent a radical resection, however in those age 85 years or more only 56% received this treatment (see **Figure 9.2** with permission from Cancer Research UK) [1].

Disease specific mortality increases from vulval cancer increases with age; women aged 50–59 years 5-year survival is 74% compared to 55% for women aged 70–89 years [1], although it should be noted when looking at overall mortality rates for vulval cancer, elderly women are significantly more likely to present with advanced disease limiting curative treatments [15].

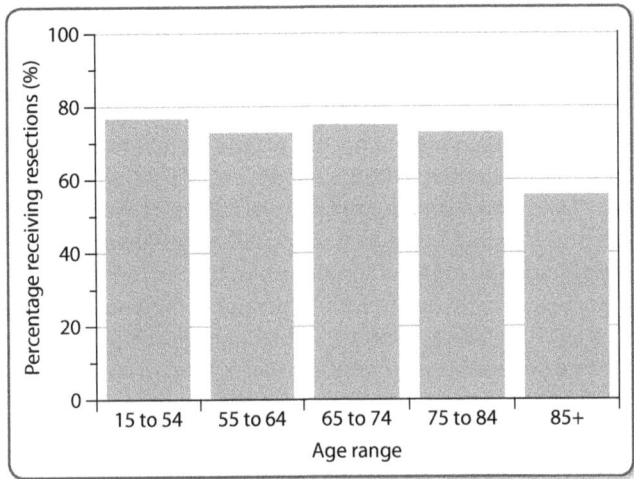

**Figure 9.2** Proportion of patients who underwent a major resection for vulval cancer by age from 2006 to 2010, in England [1].

## MANAGING ELDERLY PATIENTS WITH CANCER

Elderly patients more often have multiple co-morbidities which impact on their ability to tolerate standard treatment compared to those <65 years [10]. Although life expectancy is increasing; in the UK an 80-year-old women has an average life expectancy of 9.2 years, the numbers of years spent in 'good health' is very variable. Data from the 2011 census found in people 85 years or older only 25% described themselves of being in 'very good' or 'good' general health [13] suggesting the majority suffered from at least one significant co-morbidity impacting on their QoL.

Co-morbidities and patient choice may not however, to be the sole reasons for the large discrepancies in treatment rates (**Figure 9.2**). Healthcare professionals, family members and carers may make assumptions about an older person's preferences and evidence on the efficacies of treatments and side effects may not be available as many trials exclude older patients [10,11]. A study by National Cancer Equality Initiative/Pharmaceutical Oncology Initiative for the UK Department of Health, investigated the impact of cancer patients' age on clinicians' decision-making [11]. Although oncologists identified performance status and co-morbidities (the patient's 'biological age') as the key factors in making decisions regarding treatment for elderly patients, when they were asked to provide management plans for various cases and scenarios, the patient's chronological age appeared to influence their decisions regarding the radicality of treatment and whether curative options were chosen over and above performance status and number of co-morbidities. The overriding concern amongst oncologists was the patient's ability to tolerate the treatment and side effects as they aged. In the case of vulval cancer for stage 1b disease women aged 80 years and over are less likely to receive inguinal lymphadenectomy when compared to those aged under 50 years and more likely to receive radiotherapy [14]. Panici et al compared outcomes of women aged 75 year or more to those <75 years undergoing inguinal lymphadenectomy [16]. There was no significant difference in complication rates for each group (33%), although patients with a poor performance status were excluded from the analysis. Nodal involvement conveyed the same prognostic value in both younger and older women in terms of disease free survival and overall survival. The decision on whether to undertake an inguinal node dissection was investigated in a retrospective review of over 1000 patients in Canada [16]; older age and severe co-morbidities were the most significant factors associated with patients not undergoing groin node dissections, and age alone was given as the reason for not performing the procedure in 38% of cases (the mean age of these patients was 87 years). A further 16% of patients declined groin node dissection but reasons for this were not clear. Rauh-Hain et al found the strongest predictor of mortality from vulval cancer remains stage at presentation; however risk of death from vulval cancer increases dramatically with age when stage and grade of tumour was adjusted for; when compared to women under 50 years the mortality rate was two-fold higher for women aged 50-64 years, four-fold for those aged 65-79 years and seven-fold higher in women aged 80 years and above [14]. Data regarding patients' preferences, co-morbidities or socio-economic status, a factor well known to have a negative impact on stage of presentation and outcomes for vulval cancer in the US, was not available to the authors preventing them from taking these factors into account [18]. The study recommends in elderly women with vulval cancer clinicians need to consider 'biological or functional' age, nutritional status, co-morbidities, cognitive functioning and social support when making decisions regarding management [14]. Availability of formal and informal social support should not be underestimated and is crucial to consider when making decisions on management especially in those over 85 years of age [11].

Despite the finding of healthcare professionals possible biased attitudes based on age towards the treatment of older patients with cancer, some of the concerns regarding ability to tolerate toxicities from treatments may be well founded, with several studies reporting trends towards increased morbidity and mortality from surgery, radiotherapy and chemotherapy for elderly women with cancer including vulval disease [11,19,10]. Risk of postoperative delirium has been shown to increase [20,21] and higher rates postoperative complications such as infection, unplanned admission to critical care, longer hospital stays and requirement for discharge to nursing home facilities rather than own home have all been demonstrated in women aged 65 years or more, even those classed as 'low risk' prior to their admission [21].

Other authors however, have argued that 'full' or curative treatments should be offered to all elderly patients in order to improve outcomes [16,22]. In one retrospective study of 169 women aged 79 years or older with gynaecological malignancies, 59% of whom received 'standard' management and the remainder had partial or no treatment, those who had full treatment had improved rates of survival [22]. Partly due to its rarity, only 11% of the patients had vulval cancer and the study makes no comment regarding QoL of patients. It is also not certain whether co-morbidities influenced the survival outcomes in the group who had partial or no treatment. A further study arguing for equity in treatments offered to elderly women with gynaecological cancer is a survey assessing the attitudes of elderly women (65 years and over) to those of younger women with gynaecological malignancies [23]. This reported no difference in patient attitudes towards undergoing radical treatments, especially surgery with intent to cure. All patients answered a validated questionnaire regarding their attitudes towards cancer treatment in young and elderly patients. Elderly women felt similar to their younger counterparts that surgery with curative intent even if there was only a small chance of cure was a risk worth taking, however, in women aged 75 years and over more than two-thirds agreed with the statement 'relief from discomfort is more important than length of life'. In addition the majority of all patients (young and old) agreed 'health and happiness are more important than length of life' directly contradicting other views expressed such as 'putting up with anything to hopefully be cured of cancer' to which 82% of younger patients and 96% of those over 75 years stated they agreed with. All but one of the 189 patients in the study had a management plan in place (surgery for their disease) by the time they were recruited and were therefore a selected group; all fit enough to undergo the procedures. The answers to the survey reveal how patients themselves are often conflicted between 'the chance of cure' and the importance of 'a good quality of life'; quantity versus quality. This may be especially true in surgery for vulval cancer where treatment related side effects such as lymphoedema are relatively common and well known to have a significant negative impact on QoL [24].

## QUALITY OF LIFE AFTER TREATMENT FOR VULVAL CANCER

Although anecdotally treatment of vulval cancer is reported to have a negative impact on a woman's QoL in fact no studies investigating this subject were conducted before 2006 [24]. A longitudinal, prospective study using mixed methods including the cancer-specific European Organisation for Research on Treatment of Cancer (EORTC-QLQ-30) and the Short Form-36 (SF-36) questionnaires to assess 23 women (median age 66 years) with vulval cancer, the majority of whom underwent a triple incision vulvectomy, found physical and mental health as well as social and sexual functioning were significantly affected over the first year following treatment. Lymphoedema had the largest impact on physical functioning such as the ability to undertake activities of daily living as well as mobility. All women reported pain (postoperative, postradiotherapy or due to lymphoedema) as having a significant negative impact on many aspects of their life and for many women pain together with fatigue lasted for at least 6 months after treatment [25]. In the future sentinel node biopsy may help further to reduce some of these post-treatment side effects in selected patients and has been reported to lessen the impact on QoL in comparison to full inguinal lymphadenectomy [26]. Quality of life itself is a concept best judged by the patient themselves and making a decision regarding 'quality' versus 'quantity' may be very difficult for many patients [7] especially older patients when faced with potentially curative treatments that carry relatively high risks of short and long-term morbidity such as lymphoedema.

## TOOLS USED TO ASSIST IN MAKING TREATMENT DECISIONS

In view of the quandaries faced by both patients and clinicians in making decisions regarding treatments for cancer, attention has turned to the use of tools already commonly used in geriatric medicine to assess the health of elderly patients [27]. Although calculation of performance status is commonly used as part of the assessment of cancer patients and has shown to be very useful in younger patients at predicting a patient's ability to tolerate treatments in older patients this alone may be insufficient to predict outcomes [10]. Hyde et al found in women with vulval cancer aged 80 years or more performance status was an independent prognostic factor in predicting survival [28]; however, others suggest clinicians can be very poor at assessing a patient's ability to recovery from surgery [23].

The comprehensive geriatric assessment (CGA) has been used for many years in geriatric medicine as an approach in making an assessment of an elderly person's overall health and takes into account somatic, functional and psychological health with the aim of formulating a multidisciplinary management plan for their care [27]. A systematic review of the use of CGA in elderly patients planned for surgical treatment of their cancer found age alone did not predict postoperative outcome or complications [29]. The strongest associations with postoperative problems were poor functioning with regards to performing essential activities of daily living (washing, feeding), depression, cognitive functioning and frailty. Poorer nutritional status and polypharmacy, suggesting multiple co-morbidities, predicted longer hospital stays. Frailty, defined as unintentional weight loss, weakness, exhaustion (low physical activity and slowness of walking), was strongly associated with postoperative complications and readmission to hospital [29]. A further review studied the CGAs performance in predicting outcomes for elderly patients undergoing surgery for cancer, chemotherapy or radiotherapy [27]. For all-cause mortality following treatment frailty was the best predictor of poorer overall survival. For co-morbidities evidence was conflicting and appeared to depend on the type of scoring system used to quantify the 'severity' of co-morbidities, e.g. when the Cumulative Illness Rating Scale for Geriatrics was used the majority of studies found co-morbidities were associated with a worsening survival but the Charlson score found no association between survival and patient co-morbidities. Nutritional status and cognitive function were both found to strongly predict survival after treatment, however in contrast to the previous systematic review; depression scores and polypharmacy did not impact on overall outcomes [27,29]. Only a small number of studies have reported the use of CGA to predict toxicity to chemotherapy, completion of chemotherapy and there are no studies investigating if the use of CGA could predict the ability to tolerate radiotherapy or outcomes following radiotherapy treatment [29]. There was very little consistency between the studies included in the review in terms of the methodology or scoring systems used to assess patients. These assessments appear to be time consuming and could be quite arduous or bewildering for most patients, let alone frail elderly patients with limited cognitive functioning who have recently been diagnosed with cancer.

## PRACTICALITIES OF MANAGING ELDERLY WOMEN WITH VULVAL CANCER

Hopefully it has become clear during the chapter that the majority of patients with vulval cancer are elderly, 65 years or older, because the nature of this disease. They are, however, a very heterogeneous group; 'younger' elderly patients (65–74 years) with some co-morbidities are frequently able to tolerate standard management just as well as those under 65 years. In women over 75 years or younger patients with multiple co-morbidities additional information regarding their other medical conditions may be necessary to help individualise management plans and ensure the patient and their carers fully understand the morbidity and mortality risks of the treatment available to them. Consideration of the person's social circumstances, mental health and cognitive function as well as their physical condition must all be taken into account. These can often be challenging consultations and require the clinician to take time to explain not only standard treatments and side effects but how these may impact on the individual elderly person. Clinical nurse specialists may greatly assist in the management of these patients providing support to the patient and their family assisting them to weigh up options and make the best decisions for their treatment, as well as providing support during treatment. Preoperative assessment by an anaesthetist can also assist in decision-making especially with regards to safety of general anaesthesia and potential postoperative complications such as respiratory tract infections or cardiac events. Joint consultations with clinical oncologists allowing for discussion of alternatives to surgical treatments should be offered. Only once all of these elements have been considered and explained carefully to the patient can they make an informed choice regarding the treatment of their cancer. Some patients require longer hospital stays to ensure services are in place to allow them to go home safely and in the case of patients with cognitive impairment a best interests meeting with family members or carers is necessary before proceeding with treatment.

## CONCLUSION

The majority of women diagnosed with vulval cancer are elderly and incidence increases with age. Older women are more likely to present with more advanced disease leading to dilemmas regarding treatment options. Standard management of early stage disease is a triple incision vulvectomy, although SLN biopsy is increasingly recognised as a safe and feasible approach to reduce morbidity from groin node dissections [6].

Balancing quality and quantity of life in elderly patients with vulval cancer, especially those with multiple co-morbidities is challenging for clinicians, patients and their carers and requires all parties to take time to fully understand all treatment options and how these may impact on the woman's life.

### Key points for clinical practice

- The majority of cases of vulval cancer occur in women 70 years and over with highest rates in those 90 years or above.
- Over 90% of vulval cancers are squamous cell carcinomas.
- Lichen sclerosus is the most frequent precursor in the development of squamous cell carcinoma of the vulva in elderly women.
- Older women are more likely to present with advanced disease.
- Overall 5-year survival rates for vulval cancer 64–67%.
- Standard management of early stage disease is surgical excision of the primary tumour with disease-free margin of >8 mm, with inguinal lymph node dissection for stage 1b tumours.
- Morbidity following surgery is common; wound breakdown occurs in approximately 2040% of wide local excisions and lower limb lymphoedema after inguinal lymphadenectomy is reported in between 30–70% of cases.
- Morbidity from treatment (surgery and or radiotherapy) for vulval cancer has a significant long-term negative impact on patients' QoL.
- In elderly patients postoperative complications such as delirium may be increased with longer hospital stays and a higher risk of discharge to nursing home care rather than back to own home.
- In elderly patients, especially those 75 years or older or with multiple co-morbidities careful assessment of physical and mental health as well as cognitive functioning and social support must be undertaken before decisions regarding treatment can be made. Frailty is the biggest risk factor for poor recovery following treatment.

# REFERENCES

1. Cancer Research UK. http://www.cancerresearchuk.org/health-professional/cancer-statistics/statistics-by-cancer-type/vulval-cancer [last accessed 22.12.16]
2. Office for National Statistics June 2016. https://www.ons.gov.uk/peoplepopulationandcommunity/healthandsocialcare/conditionsanddiseases/bulletins/cancerregistrationstatisticsengland/previousReleases [last accessed 22.12.16]
3. SEER Stat Fact Sheets: Vulvar Cancer. National Cancer Institute Surveillance, Epidemiology and End Results Program. https://seer.cancer.gov/statfacts/html/vulva.html [last accessed 22.12.16]
4. Royal College of Obstetricians and Gynaecologists and British Gynaecological Cancer Society. Guidelines for the Diagnosis and Management of Vulval Carcinoma, 2014. https://www.rcog.org.uk/en/guidelines-research-services/guidelines/vulval-carcinoma-guidelines-for-the-diagnosis-and-management-of/ [last accessed 22.12.16]
5. Mutch DG. The new FIGO staging system for cancers of the vulva, cervix, endometrium and sarcomas. Gynecol Oncol 2009; 115:325–328.
6. Van der Zee AGJ, Oonk MH, De Hullu JA, et al. Sentinel node dissection is safe in the treatment of early-stage vulvar cancer. J Clin Oncol 2008; 26:884–889.
7. te Grootenhuis NC, van der Zee AG, Van Doorn HC, et al. Sentinel nodes in vulvar cancer: Long-term follow-up of the GROningen INternational Study on Sentinel nodes in Vulvar cancer (GROINSS-V) I. Gynecol Oncol 2016; 140:8–14.
8. Levenback CF, Ali S, Coleman RL, et al. Lymphatic mapping and sentinel lymph node biopsy in women with squamous cell carcinoma of the vulva: a gynecologic oncology group study. J Clin Oncol 2012; 30:3786–3791.
9. Hinten F, van den Einden LCG, Hendriks JCM, et al. Risk factors for short- and long-term complications after groin surgery in vulvar cancer. Br J Can 2011; 105:1279–1287.
10. Van Rijswijk REN, Vermorkan JB. Drug therapy for gynaecological cancer in older women. Drugs Aging 2000; 17:13–32.
11. National Cancer Equality Initiative/Pharmaceutical Oncology Initiative. The impact of patient age on clinical decision-making in oncology, 2012.
12. Kotkin J. The Changing Demographics of America. Smithsonian Magazine, 2010.
13. Office for National Statistics. Characteristics of Older People: What does the 2011 Census tell us about the "oldest old" living in England & Wales? https://www.ons.gov.uk/peoplepopulationandcommunity/birthsdeathsandmarriages/ageing/articles/characteristicsofolderpeople/2013-12-06 [last accessed 22.12.16]
14. World Health Organisation. Are you ready? What you need to know about ageing. http://www.who.int/world-health-day/2012/toolkit/background/en/index3.html [last accessed 22.12.16]
15. Rauh-Hain JA, Clemmer J, Clark RM, et al. Management and outcomes for elderly women with vulvar cancer over time. BJOG 2014; 121:719–727.
16. Panici PB, Tomao F, Domenici L, et al. Prognostic role of inguinal lymphadenectomy in vulvar squamous carcinoma: younger and older patients should be equally treated. A prospective study and literature review. Gynecol Oncol 2015; 137:373–379.
17. Gien LT, Sutradhar R, Thomas G, et al. Patient, tumor, and health system factors affecting groin node dissection rates in vulvar carcinoma: A population-based cohort study. Gynecol Oncol 2015; 139:465–470.
18. Chase DM, Lin CC, Craig CD, et al. Disparities in Vulvar Cancer Reported by the National Cancer Database: Influence of Sociodemographic Factors. Obst Gynecol 2015; 126:792–802.
19. Stuckey A, Schutzer M, Rizack T, Dizon D. Locally advanced vulvar cancer in elderly women: is chemoradiation beneficial? Am J Clin Oncol 2013; 36:279–282.
20. McAlpine JN, Hodgson EJ, Abramowitz S, et al. The incidence and risk factors associated with postoperative delirium in geriatric patients undergoing surgery for suspected gynecologic malignancies. Gynecol Oncol 2008; 109:296–302.
21. Choi J, Yoon S, Kim S, et al. Prediction of Postoperative Complications by Multidimensional Frailty Score of Older Female Cancer Patients. Gerontologist 2015; 55:529.
22. Perri T, Katz T, Korach J, et al. Treating Gynecologic Malignancies in Elderly Patients. Am J Clin Oncol 2015; 38:278–282.
23. Nordin AJ, Chinn DJ, Moloney I, et al. Do elderly cancer patients care about cure? Attitudes to radical gynecologic oncology surgery in the elderly. Gynecol Oncol 2001; 81:447–55.

24. Günthera V, Malchowb B, Schuberta M, et al. Impact of radical operative treatment on the quality of life in women with vulvar cancer – A retrospective study. Eur J Surg Oncol 2014; 40:875–882.
25. Jones GL, Jacques RM, Thompson J, et al. The impact of surgery for vulval cancer upon health-related quality of life and pelvic floor outcomes during the first year of treatment: a longitudinal, mixed methods study. Psycho-oncology 2016; 25:656–662.
26. McCann GA, Cohn DE, Jewell EL, Havrilesky LJ. Lymphatic mapping and sentinel lymph node dissection compared to complete lymphadenectomy in the management of early-stage vulvar cancer: A cost-utility analysis. Gynecol Oncol 2015; 136:300–304.
27. Hamaker ME, Vos AG, Smorenburg CH, de Rooij SE, van Munster BC. The value of Geriatric Assessments in Predicting Treatment Tolerance and All-Cause Mortality in Older Patients with Cancer. Oncologist 2012; 17:1439–1449.
28. Hyde SE, Ansink AC, Burger MPM, Schilthuis MS, van der Velden J. The Impact of Performance Status on Survival in Patients of 80 Years and Older with Vulvar Cancer Gynecol Oncol 2002; 84:388–393.
29. Feng MA, McMillan DT, Crowell K, et al. Geriatric Assessment in surgical oncology: a systematic review. J Surg Res 2015; 193:265–272.

EU GSPR Authorised Reprsentative
Logos Europe, 9 rue Nicolas Poussin
1700, La Rochelle, France
Phone: +33 (0) 6 67 93 73 78
E-mail: contact@logoseurope.eu

www.ingramcontent.com/pod-product-compliance
Ingram Content Group UK Ltd.
Pitfield, Milton Keynes, MK11 3LW, UK
UKHW051846210426
5322IPUK00019B/272